Practical Orthodontic Assessment

Practical Orthodontic Assessment

C. D. Stephens, MDS, FDSRCS Edin., FDS, MOrth RCS Eng.
Professor of Child Dental Health, University of Bristol

and

K. G. Isaacson, FDS, MOrth RCS Eng.
Consultant Orthodontist, Oxford Regional Health Authority

Heinemann Medical Books

Heinemann Medical Books
An imprint of Heinemann Professional Publishing Ltd
Halley Court, Jordan Hill, Oxford OX2 8EJ

OXFORD LONDON SINGAPORE NAIROBI
IBADAN KINGSTON

First published 1990

British Library Cataloguing in Publication Data
Stephens, C. D.
Practical orthodontic assessment.
1. Dentistry. Orthodontics
I. Title II. Isaacson, K. G. (Keith Geoffrey)
617.6′43

ISBN 0 433 00064 3

Filmset by Eta Services (Typesetters) Ltd, Beccles, Suffolk
Printed in Great Britain by Thomson Litho, East Kilbride, Glasgow

Contents

Preface

Over the years, despite greater availability of good orthodontic textbooks and a general improvement in undergraduate teaching, the constant demand in all the undergraduate and postgraduate orthodontic courses we have run has been for more practice in treatment planning. This is perhaps not surprising. In orthodontics treatment planning may still begin with the treat/do not treat decision but thereafter a multiplicity of interrelated factors must be taken into account. When should the case be treated? Is ideal treatment realistic or should a less ambitious alternative be accepted? Do teeth need to be removed – if so, which? What mechanics are required to achieve the desired tooth movements? What anchorage is necessary for the appliances to be used and how will this be provided? What retention is required at the end of treatment and what is the prognosis for stability after appliances are withdrawn?

This book is designed to meet such a need. We are aware that in attempting this we have laid ourselves open to a variety of criticisms from both practitioners and our specialist colleagues. Clearly 20 cases are insufficient to cover all but a tiny sample of treatment planning decisions. We have also been limited by the number of illustrations which could be included. Some of the results are not ideal but we felt it dishonest to pretend that even in our hands the correct treatment plan always produces perfect results.

Many of the cases we have included only go to show that the complexity of the treatment is beyond that which a general practitioner should attempt. Some might consider this to be wasted space and of no interest to the general dental practitioner, but recent examination of the results of practitioner orthodontics has shown us that such cases are frequently attempted in a mistaken belief that they can be satisfactorily treated with maxillary removable appliances.

We would welcome any comments readers may wish to make.

Acknowledgements

We wish to acknowledge the generous assistance of J. J. Thompson, Orthodontic Laboratories of Sheffield in the preparation of the plaster models used in this book.

Thanks are also due to Mr S Adams BDS who digitized the cephalometric radiographs and to Mr N Isaacson who prepared the tracings.

SECTION ONE

Case assessment and treatment planning

CHAPTER 1
How to carry out orthodontic case assessment

INTRODUCTION

Many readers will already have their own scheme of examining orthodontic patients. However the layout of this book means that the user is virtually obliged to follow strictly the examination scheme as outlined here (and summarized in the inside cover) since the definitive assessment of each case will be given in this order. Whilst the particular regime we have adopted is probably no better than any other, it has been evolved during 20 years of clinical teaching and has been subject to modification in the light of experience and of comments from colleagues.

The assessment of the potential orthodontic patient follows the same general pattern as all other dental examinations: firstly, the history and secondly, the examination.

It is probably best to devote two appointments to the orthodontic assessment because it is difficult if not impossible to reach firm conclusions about treatment (as opposed to decision on the need for treatment) without the aid of study models.

At the first visit a dental and medical history should be obtained. An idea of the patients likely interest in orthodontic treatment should be assessed; if this is favourable, impressions for reference models should be taken together with up-to-date radiographs (see below). Both the extraoral and intraoral examination should be delayed until study models have been prepared.

THE HISTORY

Medical history

Fortunately very few medical conditions preclude the wearing of appliances. In those children with a history of poorly controlled epilepsy, treatment should be delayed until a suitable anticonvulsant regime has been established. Those patients with heart conditions, blood dyscrasias and patients on drug regimes such as steroids or chemotherapeutic agents may need special management if extractions are required.

Dental history

Because the enthusiastic support of both parent and patient are required if orthodontic treatment is to be successfully carried out, it is essential to obtain a history which includes the views of both child and parent. What are they concerned about? Do they understand what orthodontic treatment involves? Have other children in the family successfully completed treatment? How far away do they live? Do they attend school locally? Does the family have a car? If not how reliable is public transport? How easy is it to have time off school? Clearly if you are seeing the patient for routine treatment most of these answers will have been obtained at earlier visits. But if the patient is not well known to you we advise that you should see him or her alone at some point during this second visit to establish the child's own views independently of parental interjection.

EXTRAORAL EXAMINATION

A systematic approach is essential. If the same set pattern is always followed then nothing will be left out. This is particularly important in what is largely an elective form of treatment.

The extraoral examination falls into two parts:

1 It is necessary first to identify the skeletal framework upon which the dentoalveolar processes have developed.
2 Then the muscular environment which envelops them must be observed and recorded.

It is true to say that whilst a severe skeletal discrepancy always has a highly significant bearing on the treatment plan, it is seldom the case that the soft tissue form or behaviour dictates the treatment. However it will affect the prognosis and may influence a decision about whether treatment should be attempted.

By the time the intraoral examination is undertaken the experienced practitioner should already have some idea about the type of occlusion one would expect to see. Indeed it is important that he or she should attempt to visualize this for if the relationship of the dental arches does not correspond with the clinician's expectations this implies that the extraoral assessment or its interpretation is incorrect. For example, a Class 1 skeletal pattern and competent soft tissues should produce a Class I incisor relationship. If this is not the case than some other contributory factor must be identified.

Skeletal form

Anteroposterior jaw relationship (skeletal class)
This part of the examination is best carried out with the patient seated upright in the dental chair with the head in the free postural position, that is, looking straight ahead with the eyes directed at the

horizon. Usually the Frankfort plane will also be approximately horizontal when in this posture (Fig. 1.1). The face is examined in profile to assess the anteroposterior relationship of the basal parts of the jaws to each other. It is usually much easier to make this assessment standing a little way back from the patient. Ideally the maxillary base should lie about 2 or 3 mm anterior to the mandibular base when the teeth are in occlusion (Fig. 1.1). It may be difficult to be certain of this relationship by merely looking at the anterior contour of the face when the jaws are still covered by the lips. Minor variations from the ideal may not be of any consequence; however, any marked discrepancy seen at this stage will usually indicate that its correction is probably beyond the scope of the general practitioner.

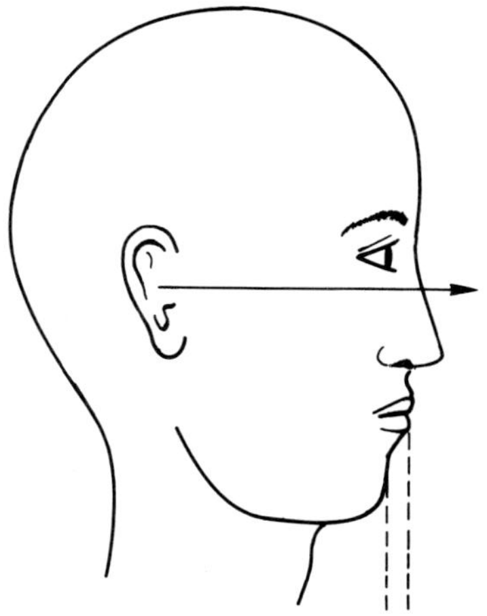

Fig. 1.1

For the mild case, a better idea of the skeletal class may be gained by retracting the lips and observing the relationship of the labial plates of bone overlying the apices of the upper and lower central incisor teeth. Usually this is best carried out indirectly by palpating the areas of concavity in the labial plates and estimating the relationship of one's fingertips. Some authorities have suggested that by using the index and second finger the angulation of the hand gives an indication of the skeletal class. If the hand is level it is Class 1. If the wrist is elevated (with the hand angled down) it is Class 3, and if the hand points upwards it is Class 2. Note that the skeletal class relates upper and lower apical bases to each other and not to the face. In other words, the classification 'skeletal 2' does not reveal whether the mandible is 'too far back' or the maxilla 'too far forwards' (Fig. 1.2).

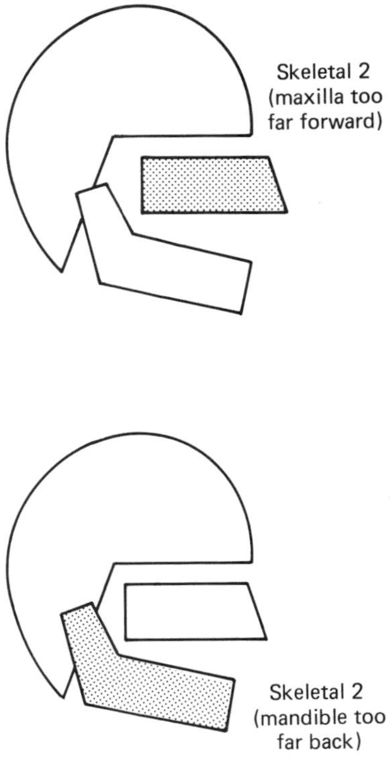

Fig. 1.2

In this text we have included a lateral skull tracing for the interest of those who are familiar with this clinical aid. For those who are not, assessment can be made based on the soft tissue outline and the outline of the labial plates of bone overlying the upper and lower incisor roots.

Vertical relationship (lower face height)
With the face still in profile and the teeth in occlusion, an estimate should be made of the lower face height. This should be done both as a linear distance and as a proportion of the total face height. Does the lower part of the face appear excessively long or short? Usually the distance from a point between the eyebrows to the junction of the nose with the upper lip will be roughly equal to the distance from below the nose to the underside of the chin. Usually reduced lower face heights are associated with deep overbites whilst excessive lower face heights may be the cause of anterior open bites. The latter are called 'skeletal' open bites to distinguish them from those of soft tissue aetiology.

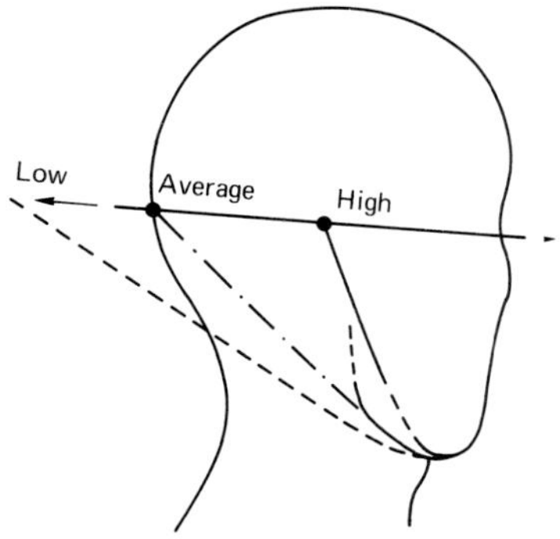

Fig. 1.3

In addition you should estimate the angle between the Frankfort and mandibular planes (Fig 1.3). Increased face heights are seen where this angle is raised and vice versa. However because of the difficulty of judging angles it is more reliable to use the location of the point of intersection of these two planes rather than the angle between them.

Lateral relationship (facial asymmetry)
Very few faces are truly symmetrical. Facial asymmetry may be the result of biological variation, pathology or congenital abnormality. Fortunately, because the alveolar processes are moulded by the enveloping soft tissues, even quite marked asymmetry of the lower part of the face frequently fails to produce a disturbance in the occlusion of the teeth. Nevertheless asymmetry should be checked for. Even if it appears to be of no significance it should be regularly reviewed in the growing child as such conditions may become progressively worse. Where the occlusion is affected this will usually be in the form of a buccal crossbite – a disturbance in the relationship of the buccal teeth in the coronal plane such that the palatal cusps of the upper teeth no longer occlude in the fossae of their antagonists.

Asymmetry in the lower part of the face can arise in two ways. Either the face itself is asymmetrical or the patient may have adopted a displaced path of mandibular closure to avoid a premature contact as the teeth are brought into occlusion.

During the extraoral examination the patient should have adopted a relaxed posture and unless instructed otherwise will adopt a resting mandibular posture. Observe the patient's face from above and slightly behind. Does the midpoint of the chin coincide with the mid-facial plane? If not, is it the upper or lower face which is at fault?

Whilst discussing lateral relationships of the jaws, mention should be made of the width of the arches. Usually that of the upper jaw will be similar to that of the lower. Occasionally one jaw is very much wider than the other, to such an extent that the occlusal relationships of the buccal teeth are affected and a buccal crossbite is seen. As there are other much more common causes of crossbite it is only necessary to bear this aetiology in mind when the intraoral examination reveals the presence of a bilateral buccal crossbite.

Soft tissue form and behaviour

The lips

As the dental base determines the position of the apices of the teeth, so the form and action of the lips and tongue are largely responsible for the positions of the crowns of the teeth. We are interested in assessing lip contour, lip competence and lip line.

Lip contour—In profile, with the patient sitting upright and relaxed, are the lips everted, (in which case the underlying teeth might be expected to be proclined) or are they rather vertical with no obvious outward curve at the red margin? The average lies between these two extremes (Fig. 1.4).

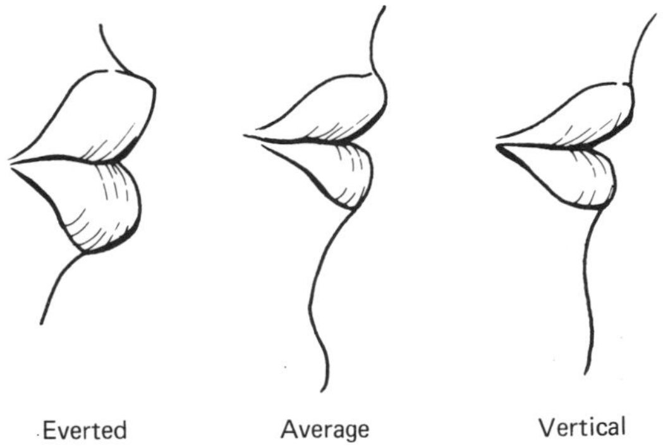

Fig. 1.4

Lip competence—Do the lips form a seal at rest or are they too short to do this when the mandible is also in its resting position (lip incompetence)? Many individuals with mild lip incompetence unconsciously hold their lips together by slight circumoral contraction for a significant portion of the time and this is difficult to detect. The tell-tale signs are a flattening out of the submental fold of the lower lip and a slight dimpling over the anterior surface of the chin where the fibres of the mentalis muscle are inserted.

Lip line—Where is the crest of the lower lip with respect to the upper incisor tips (Fig. 1.5). Although this is referred to as the lip line, it is applied only to the relationship of the lower lip to the upper (central) incisors. Ideally, at rest, the lower lip covers between a third and a half of the labial surface of the upper central incisors. In a Class II division 1 malocclusion the lip line will be lower and often fail to control the upper incisors, whilst in a Class II division 2 incisor relationship it will be much higher, sometimes covering the entire labial surface of the crown.

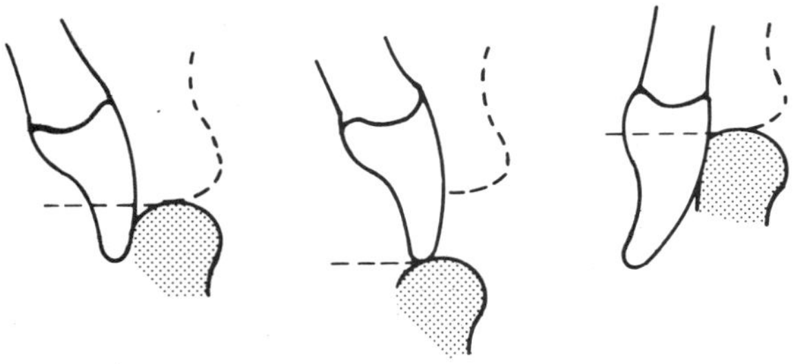

Fig. 1.5

Clinical observation suggests that the presence of the lower lip labial to the tip of the upper incisors is largely responsible for maintaining a treated Class II division 1 malocclusion. This appears to be less true when fixed appliances are used and ideal incisal and interincisal angulations can be obtained, but crucial where removable appliances are employed. In Class I and II division 2 incisor relationships the upper incisors are already 'within lip control' and the assessment of soft tissue form and behaviour is of less significance. Fortunately the desire to maintain a lip seal appears to increase until the late teens and so some quite unfavourable lip forms manage to retain corrected Class II division 1 incisor occlusions. Nevertheless such cases should be given a rather guarded prognosis where removable appliances are to be used or referred for more complex treatment.

The tongue

Tongue behaviour is even more difficult to assess. In the past a great deal of time was spent classifying the behaviour of the tongue at rest and during swallowing.

It is to be expected that where the lips are incompetent the tongue will be used to produce a seal at the front of the mouth during swallowing. This can sometimes be demonstrated by pulling the lower lip downward and forward at the moment of swallowing and revealing the tip of the tongue interposed between the incisors. This 'adaptive' lip–tongue–palate seal is probably used because it requires less effort than a seal produced by drawing the lips together. Not surprisingly, it is more commonly seen in Class II division 1 malocclusion where the upper incisors make circumoral contraction more difficult. At other times in such cases the tongue may lie resting on the lower incisors, where it may prevent the full vertical development of the anterior dentoalveolar processes, leading to an incomplete overbite.

The adaptive tongue to lower lip seal tends to disappear as dental development proceeds, particularly if a Class II division 1 incisor occlusion is corrected. Not too much importance should be attached to adaptive tongue thrusts. Very occasionally tongue thrusting appears to be part of an inbuilt pattern of neuromuscular behaviour. These endogenous tongue thrusts, which account for less than 1% of all thrusts, cannot be changed by treatment. It is therefore highly desirable to distinguish between the two types of tongue thrust. Unfortunately this is not always possible but signs to beware of are:

1 Proclination of both upper and lower incisors.
2 An absence of lip incompetence associated with the thrust.
3 Presence of a large part of the tongue between the anterior teeth at all times.
4 A reversed curve of Spee in both arches.
5 A marked lisp.

Finally, mention should be made of the effects of digit-sucking habits which often cause the tongue to come to lie between the teeth and occupy the space which the thumb or finger has vacated. The effect which the thumb has is very variable and the severity of the habit at the time of examination has little bearing on the incisor malocclusion.

INTRAORAL EXAMINATION

The recommended procedure for your examination, which will be used in subsequent sections of this book is as follows:

1 Obtain a general idea of the condition of the mouth.
2 Examine each arch separately, looking in turn at the incisors, canines and buccal teeth.
3 Examine the teeth in occlusion and record the occlusal relationships of each segment to its opponent in the same order.

General condition of the mouth

- First count the teeth.
- Is the plaque control adequate for active treatment?
- Do the restorations appear to be of good quality?
- Are any teeth hypoplastic or of unusual form or size?
- Are there any periodontal problems such as a Stilman's cleft associated with a traumatized lower incisor?

Then examine each arch in turn, as follows.

Examination of the lower arch

Labial segment

Are the lower incisors acceptably aligned, spaced or crowded? If crowded, some attempt should be made to grade this: mild, moderate, and severe are usually sufficient. Are any teeth bodily displaced from the arch? Are any teeth rotated with respect to the line of the arch or is any crowding merely labiolingual displacement? It is customary to describe rotations by identifying the corner of the incisal edge which is most displaced from the arch and indicating the direction in which it is displaced, hence: mesiolabial, distolingual

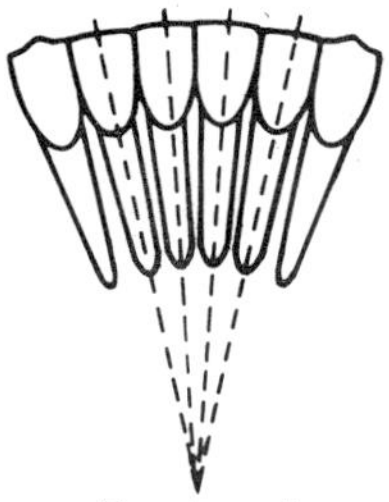

Fanning of lower incisors

Fig. 1.6

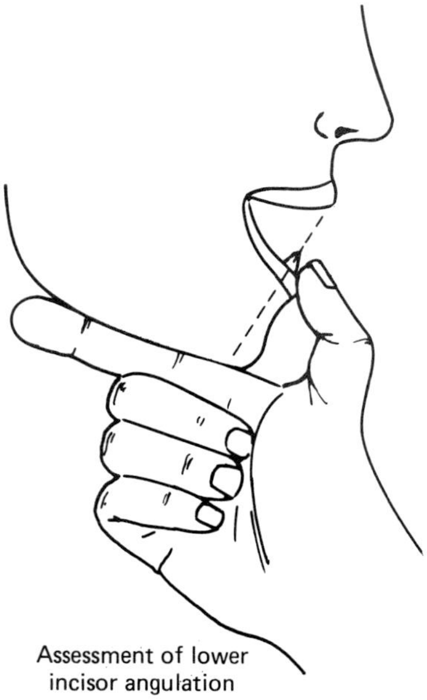

Assessment of lower incisor angulation

Fig. 1.7

etc. Are any teeth significantly tilted mesially or distally? Sometimes all the lower incisors appear to be splayed distally – aptly referred to as 'fanning' (Fig. 1.6). The incisor centreline must be checked for its relationship to the mid-plane of the face.

It is also important to estimate the angulation of the lower labial teeth with the lower border of the mandible. This will help to confirm your estimate of the form and behaviour of the lips. Usually the lower incisors are set at about 90° to the lower border. Any marked difference should be noted. You will find it helpful to place your index finger along the lower border of the mandible and, retracting the lip with the thumb of the same hand, view the patient from the side to make this estimate (Fig. 1.7).

Finally check the gingival margins to ensure that they have an adequate zone of attached gingiva. This is particularly important where there is a labially crowded incisor. If this is less than 1 mm a more thorough examination of the fraenal and muscle attachments in this region should be made. (This will not be possible from the records presented in Section Two but where appropriate a clinical note will be added to the pretreatment records.)

Canines

The examination of each canine area should be made in turn. Is there sufficient space to accommodate each tooth? Where crowding exists the canine will usually be excluded buccally and if unerupted should be seen as a bulge. Partial eruption and supraeruption should be recorded. The angulation of the erupted canine has an important bearing on treatment planning (mesially inclined teeth can be retracted with removable appliances; upright or distally inclined canines usually require a fixed appliance). This angle should be estimated with respect to the occlusal plane and the inclination of each canine classified as mesial, upright or distal. Any rotation is described in the same way as for incisors.

Buccal segments

In the established permanent dentition the degree of crowding may be easily estimated and should be recorded either in millimetres or as a fraction of a premolar width (hence one-third of a unit crowding etc.). Frequently at the time of the orthodontic examination the deciduous molars will still be retained and it may be difficult to estimate the degree of crowding in the buccal segments. On the other hand where a deciduous molar has been lost prematurely, and the successional tooth is unerupted, an estimate of the crowding can sometimes be made using the dimension of a contralateral premolar as a guide. Remember that apart from the third molars, second premolars are the most common teeth to be congenitally absent. They are also frequently hypoplastic. If second premolars are crowded through early loss they will usually be displaced lingually and delayed in their eruption. It is unusual to be able to palpate a lingually displaced premolar much before 13 or 14 years of age. Where teeth are rotated these should be noted.

Examination of the upper arch

Incisors

This examination is carried out in an identical manner to that for the lower incisor teeth; the only difference is that the angulation of upper incisor teeth is recorded with respect to the Frankfort plane. Remember that supernumerary teeth are common in this region of the mouth and may cause displacement, rotation or non-eruption of a permanent maxillary central incisor. A naso-occlusal radiograph is advisable even if the region appears to be normal. Orthopantomographic x-rays do not give a sufficiently clear picture of the upper incisor region and must be supplemented with an occlusal or intraoral view.

Deciduous and permanent central incisors are also frequently subjected to trauma. Fractured incisors are obvious, dilacerations less so. Remember to note the presence of any white patches, areas of decalcification or discoloration on the labial surfaces of anterior teeth. It is important to bring these to the parents' attention before treatment is carried out. Where necessary, tests should be made for vitality.

Lateral incisors are frequently congenitally absent but they may also be crowded palatal to the line of the arch. Where one lateral incisor is congenitally absent the contralateral tooth may well be rather small or 'peg-shaped'. Palatal invaginations are also common: remember to check both radiographically and clinically for these.

Canines

The examination of each canine should be made as for the lower arch. Where the canine is unerupted it will usually be palpable buccally, particularly if it is rather short of space. Unfortunately the maxillary canine is often misplaced and this possibility should be confirmed or excluded as early as possible. If by $10\frac{1}{2}$ years of age the canine cannot be palpated high up in the buccal sulcus, check to exclude the possibility that it is palatally misplaced. The angulation of the erupted lateral incisor will often give a clue as to the likely position of the canine. Check also to see if the deciduous canine (or the permanent lateral) is mobile. If necessary, localizing radiographs must be taken (see above). The earlier this problem can be identified, the easier will be its treatment.

Buccal segments

This examination is carried out precisely as for the lower arch. Estimate the degree of crowding and note its location.

The examination of the teeth in occlusion

Path of closure

As the teeth are brought into contact the mandible should make a simple hinge movement from its resting position with the condyles rotating in their glenoid fossae. Not infrequently, either as a result of dental crowding or skeletal discrepancy, two teeth meet prematurely. The mandible then makes a lateral or forward displacement from its path of closure. (If a displacement is present in one of the exercise cases this will be mentioned.) Whether a displacement is found or not, all assessments of incisor and buccal occlusal relationships should be made with the teeth fully intercuspated.

Incisor occlusion

Overjet—Measure this from the labial surface of the lower incisor to the labial surface of the upper incisor. Record the distance for both central incisors. Get used to making the measurement in the middle of each incisal edge, keeping the ruler parallel to the occlusal plane. With practice this can be accurately estimated by eye to within a millimetre, even from non-scale photographs – try it!

Overbite—Clinically this can be assessed by measurement of models. (In this text the labial photograph of the model does not always permit the overbite to be ascertained. We suggest you use the lateral skull where the overbite is deep and the crown of the lower incisors cannot be seen on the models.) Terms used to describe overbite are:

Increased (more than 4 mm)
Reduced (less than 3 mm)
Complete (the lower incisor tips touch opposing tooth or mucosa)
Incomplete (the lower incisor tips fail to meet the opposing tooth or mucosa).

Incisor class—This is based on the anatomy of the palatal contour of the incisor crown (Fig. 1.8). A common error is to forget that in the child only part of the full clinical crown is in the mouth. Many Class I incisor occlusions are identified incorrectly as Class II division 1 relationships for this reason.

Centrelines—Do these coincide? If not, which is incorrect. Check by looking down from above and behind the patient in the same way as you did for facial asymmetry. If there is a centreline shift in the lower arch, check to see if this is due to a mandibular displacement.

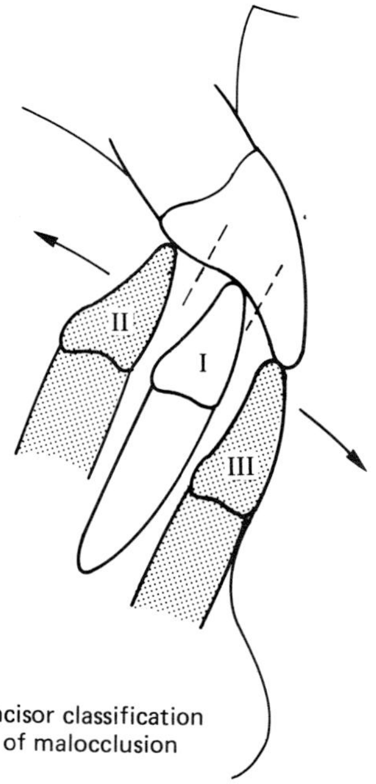

Incisor classification of malocclusion

Fig. 1.8

Canine occlusion
With the teeth together the occlusion of the canines is classified. Usually this will correlate with the buccal occlusion (see Fig. 1.9) but where there has been early loss or if there are differing degrees of crowding in the two arches this will not be the case (see below).

Buccal segments

Buccal occlusion—The anteroposterior occlusion of the buccal teeth should be classified as shown in Figure 1.9. Note that a distinction is made between half-unit discrepancies where the teeth occlude cusp to cusp and full unit discrepancies. The unit referred to is the width

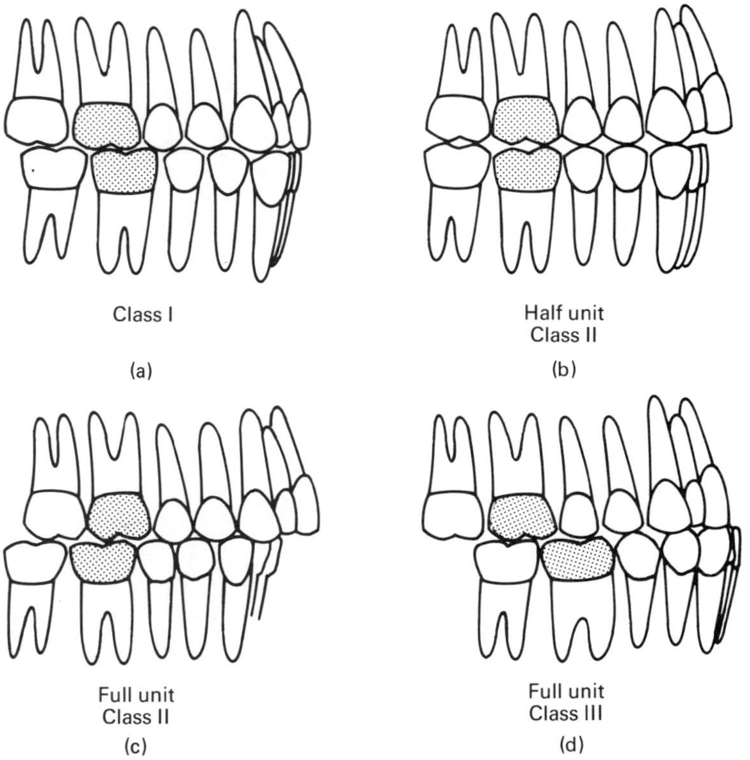

Fig. 1.9

of a premolar. Generally the whole buccal segment will have the same type of occlusion and one can note that 'the left buccal segment is a full unit Class II'. If there has been premature loss of deciduous teeth the canine and molar occlusion will be different and it may be necessary to record molar and canine occlusion separately (Fig. 1.10).

Crossbites—Where the teeth occlude with the buccal cusps of the lower teeth outside (buccal to) those of the upper teeth, a crossbite is said to exist. Crossbites may affect just one tooth (typically an upper second premolar following early loss) and are described as local. Almost invariably they are due to crowding – for example the crowded upper second premolar mentioned above.

Segmental crossbites, on the other hand, affect most of the buccal teeth and may be unilateral or bilateral. They are due to a discrepancy in the width of one arch to the other which may be dento-alveolar or skeletal in origin. For example, a digit-sucking habit is frequently the cause of a unilateral posterior crossbite. Unilateral crossbites are usually associated with a mandibular displacement which should be checked for (see above). Bilateral crossbites are rarely caused by soft tissue influences and are usually the expression of a discrepancy in the width of the dental bases – in other words, skeletal in origin.

In the UK crossbites are described in terms of the position of the lower teeth with respect to the upper. This is very strange because the width of the lower arch usually cannot be changed. Hence a

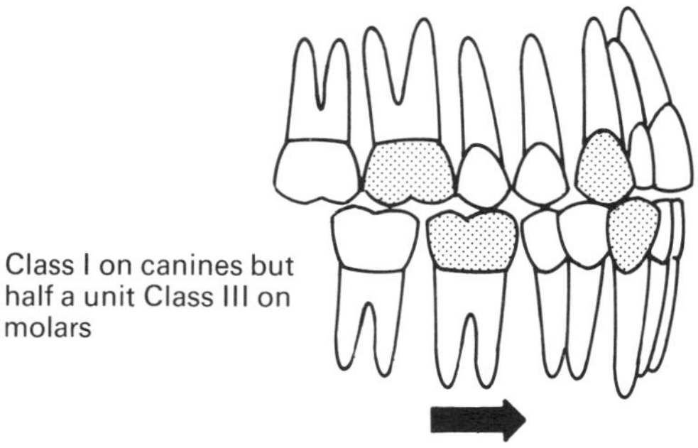

(a)

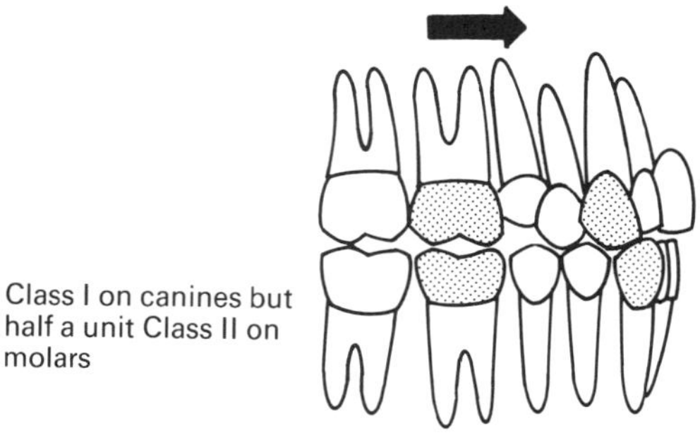

(b)

Fig. 1.10

unilateral left buccal crossbite means that the lower teeth are buccal to the upper ones on that side. In the USA the same term would mean that the lingual cusps of the upper posterior teeth were occluding completely buccal to the buccal cusps of the lower.

THE EXAMINATION OF RADIOGRAPHS

Like the rest of your examination, this must be done systematically. It is absolutely essential to confirm the presence and good prognosis of all teeth before elective extractions are planned. Count the teeth in each quadrant from anterior to posterior. Look first at the crowns, identifying each tooth in turn and examining the crown and pulp chamber. Although extraoral films are not ideal for diagnosing caries it is surprising how frequently cavities are seen. Next look at the roots of each tooth for unusual form (dilaceration, internal or external resorption etc.). Finally examine the surrounding bone, both locally immediately around the tooth and more distantly. On the orthopantomogram this should include maxillary sinuses and condyles.

CHAPTER 2

How to plan orthodontic treatment

PRINCIPLES

It is important to recognize that a large number of malocclusions do not require treatment on the grounds of dental health. Hence if the patient is unconcerned about the malocclusion it is acceptable in many instances to advise that no treatment should be undertaken. This is particularly true of the mild malocclusion where any real improvement requires an ideal occlusion to be obtained. This is really only possible if fixed appliances are used competently, the patient co-operates fully with treatment and nothing relapses after appliances are withdrawn.

On the other hand, occasionally the clinician will come across grossly disfiguring malocclusions which parents feel are quite acceptable. We have all heard comments such as 'I hope my daughter will never have to depend upon her looks to make her way in the world'. Such peculiarly British sentiments are rather difficult to deal with but where the patient has been seen initially without the parent and has stated quite clearly his or her concern about the malocclusion, it is sometimes possible to convince the parent of the need for treatment.

Situations where orthodontic treatment is indicated on dental health grounds generally include the following:

1 Traumatic occlusion, where damage can be seen to be occurring.
2 Excessive overjets where these are sufficient to place the upper anterior at risk through accidental damage. Such a situation depends to a large extent on the lip cover but is usually taken as being overjets of 7 mm and more.
3 A crossbite associated with a mandibular displacement.
4 Severe crowding.
5 Impacted and unerupted teeth.
6 Where tooth movement is required to facilitate some other aspect of dentistry, for example periodontal splinting.

TIMING OF TREATMENT

The age of 10–14 years is usually regarded as the optimum time for most orthodontic treatment. By this time the greater part of facial growth has taken place; the relationship of the arches is established and will be unlikely to change significantly.

However, at this age most children still have some facial growth to take place which will be accompanied by compensatory tooth eruption. Hence overbite reduction and spontaneous tooth movements will still occur quite readily in most cases. Increasing social awareness in children of this age leads to good motivation, although by 14 years co-operation may become less certain.

Early treatment

There is no evidence that orthodontic treatment in the deciduous dentition is any more long-lasting than the deciduous teeth themselves. With the eruption of the permanent incisors limited treatment can be of advantage in the correction of crossbites (particularly anterior crossbites where there is any evidence of gingival damage). Other treatment which may be indicated in the period 6–10 years includes the management of unerupted or grossly ectopic teeth and immediate measures which may be required in the event of traumatic loss of maxillary incisors or enforced extraction of deciduous molars.

Late treatment

After 14 years treatment becomes progressively more difficult. Growth is limited and hence spontaneous changes are less likely to occur. In addition co-operation may well leave a great deal to be desired. The range of cases which can be successfully treated with removable appliances in this age group is therefore reduced.

Adult treatment

Except where very minor tooth movement is being undertaken (for example, prior to prosthetic or crown and bridge work) adult orthodontics should, in our view, be seen as the province of the specialist.

THE STAGES OF TREATMENT PLANNING

To treat or not to treat?

Decide whether treatment is indicated on dental health or aesthetic grounds.

Ideal or compromise

It is better to achieve a compromise result than to fail to achieve an ideal result. There may be patients who by reason of the distance they have to travel may not be able to receive ideal specialist treatment. It is essential however that a compromise treatment does confer benefit and does not leave the patient worse off in the long term.

Space requirements

Lower arch first

Look at the lower arch to decide whether extractions are indicated or whether the alignment is acceptable. It is necessary to allow for posterior crowding and for the fact that lower arch crowding gets significantly worse with growth. This change is particularly marked during the pubertal growth of boys of 13–16 years. In cases which are suitable for treatment by the general dental practitioner the labiolingual position of the lower incisors should not be deliberately altered. Where there is moderate lower incisor crowding in a growing patient, instanding or labially placed incisors can be expected to align spontaneously following extraction of premolars for the relief of crowding. On the other hand any appliance which might advance the lower labial segment or expand the lower intercanine distance should be avoided since such changes are not stable in the majority of cases.

Upper arch

In order to have enough space to reduce any overjet and relieve crowding, the easiest guide is to ensure that there is enough room (with or without extraction) to retract the upper canines into their correct Class I articulation with their opponents. Allowance has to be made for any pre-existing crowding in the lower labial segment. This means imagining where the lower canines will be when any lower incisor crowding has been relieved before matching the position of the upper canines to these corrected positions. Clearly this guide only applies if all teeth in the labial segments are present and of normal size – beware of missing lower incisors and small upper lateral incisors.

Matching of extraction sites

Because space closure is easier to achieve if the buccal teeth can come forward together, it is usually desirable to keep extraction sites in the lower arch matched by similar extractions in the upper arch. In other words, *keep extraction sites opposite each other* (Fig. 2.1). This is not invariably the case and where fixed appliances are to be used (which will control the tendency of unopposed teeth to overerupt) other factors such as the needs of anchorage may take precedence. It perhaps hardly needs to be said that if there is no need for extractions in the lower arch, the question of keeping extraction sites opposed in this way does not arise. However where removable appliances are to be used extraction of lower first premolars will almost always dictate that the upper first premolars are the teeth of choice.

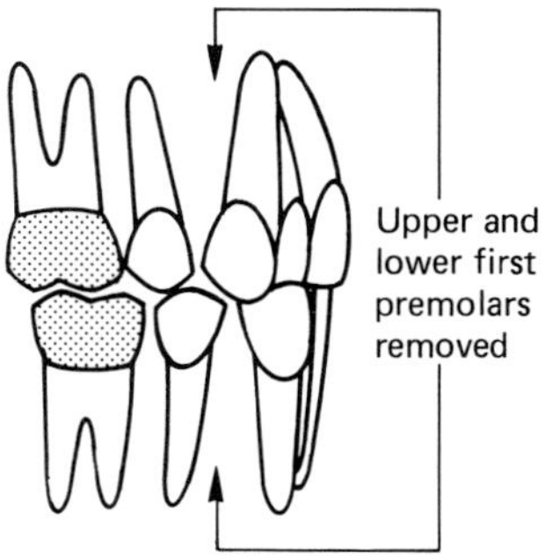

Fig. 2.1

Tooth movements required

It is best to list the precise movements required and then to determine whether the case requires appliances and whether these are of the fixed or removable type.

Spontaneous changes
Mesially inclined canines will usually spontaneously drop distally to some extent once space is available provided they are still erupting and that there is no occlusal interference. This tendency is especially marked in the lower arch but declines rapidly in the first few months after extraction. Certainly it is unusual to see any significant change beyond 6 months post-extraction. Although lower incisors tend to follow such canine alignment, do not expect rotated lower incisors to improve. It is only labiolingual displacements which can be relied on to do so.

In the upper arch spontaneous alignment of crowded incisors is minimal. The only other change which can be relied upon is the tendency for extraction spaces to close. Despite frequent talk of 'dumping' and 'collapse' into extraction spaces, provided a good molar occlusion is established first, premolar space closure achieved in this way is accomplished with minimal changes in the axial changes of the adjacent teeth. It must be remembered that this is a growth-related change and that in the post-pubertal patient (after 14 years in girls and 16 years in boys), such space closure will be very slow to take place.

Removable appliances—These are suitable for tipping movements so the axial inclination of teeth adjacent to extraction sites should be carefully assessed. Will the tipping of these teeth towards the extraction site lead to an acceptable contact area being established? Where the upper incisors are to be retracted (or in the case of Class III occlusion, advanced), will they achieve an acceptable angulation both within the face and to the opposing arch (interincisal angle)? Provided they are worn conscientiously, upper removable appliances are very effective space maintainers and are particularly appropriate for the case where upper premolars have been removed to allow a buccally crowded canine to improve as it erupts. In such cases it is then a simple matter to add a spring should complete alignment not be achieved spontaneously.

A removable appliance carrying an anterior bite plane is very effective at reducing excessive overbites in the growing patient and posterior bite planes are favoured for the elimination of mandibular displacing activity concurrently with correction of an instanding incisor or maxillary expansion to eliminate a unilateral posterior crossbite.

Functional appliances—These are particularly useful in the early correction of selected Class II division 1 cases. However because of the ease with which these appliances procline the lower incisors, we do not advise their use by general practitioners unless they have received further postgraduate training and they have access to consultant advice and cephalometric radiography.

Fixed appliances—Rotations, bodily retraction of teeth, space closure, extrusion and intrusion of individual teeth all require fixed appliances. It is also usually advisable to use fixed appliances where there are a large number of individual tooth movements to be undertaken. This is because whilst several removable appliances would be required to undertake these, the same fixed appliance can often achieve all of them. Furthermore usually many of the movements can be undertaken simultaneously when fixed appliances are used.

Surgery—Minor surgical procedures may be required in the management of displaced and unerupted teeth. Major orthognathic surgery is now routinely used in the correction of gross vertical and horizontal discrepancies. In general such treatment will require preparatory tooth alignment using fixed appliances and will not be undertaken until facial growth is complete.

Plan the buccal occlusion

Molar occlusion does not change spontaneously, hence this must be taken into account in the treatment plan. In the intact ideal occlusion there are the same number of teeth in each quadrant and the incisor occlusion is Class I, as is the molar occlusion. For this reason, if no extractions are to be undertaken, or the same number of teeth are to be removed in all quadrants, and a class I incisor occlusion is to be obtained at the end of treatment, steps must also be taken to obtain (or preserve) a Class I molar occlusion (see Fig. 2.1). If, on the other hand, only upper first premolars are to be removed the molar occlusion must end up a full unit Class II if there is to be no excess space in the upper arch at the end of treatment (Fig. 2.2).

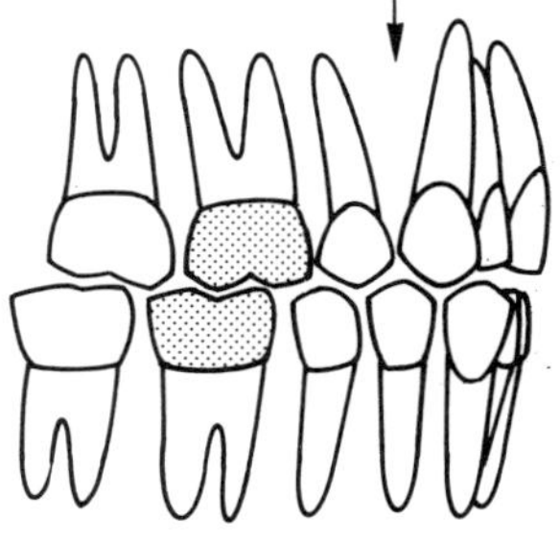

Fig. 2.2

Plan anchorage

If more than half the space provided by the removal of an upper first premolar unit is required for the alignment of anterior teeth then headgear will be required to reinforce the anchorage. (In making this estimation remember to allow for any distal retraction which will have to be made in the lower arch to permit the lower incisors to align or be aligned – see above.) In a Class II case extraoral anchorage is almost always required either to move upper buccal teeth distally to make space or to obtain a Class I molar relationship.

Design your appliances

See below.

Plan retention

See below

REMOVABLE APPLIANCE DESIGN

Before designing the appliance it goes without saying that a treatment plan has been drawn up listing the required tooth movements and the order in which these are to be carried out.

General principles

1 In general for reasons of anchorage only two single rooted teeth should be moved at any time.
2 Two active elements per appliance are best. Four should only be included in exceptional circumstances. This is not to say that appliances cannot be modified during treatment to avoid remaking the appliance unnecessarily.
3 Where only just sufficient space exists to carry out the required tooth movement, reinforcement of the anchorage with headgear is obligatory. In other cases, if in doubt make provision for extraoral anchorage. In a typical premolar extraction case half the extraction space will be lost unless extraoral anchorage is being employed.
4 Active elements in decreasing order of preference are: palatal springs – buccal springs – screws – elastics.
5 There should only be one wire crossing each contact point (there is not room for more).
6 Soldered joints should be avoided if at all possible.
7 Lower removable appliances are of very limited use. They can be successfully employed in two situations:
   (a) in the retraction of mesially inclined mandibular canines.
   (b) in the unilateral distal movement of a molar.

STEPS IN APPLIANCE DESIGN

Step 1

Choose the active element for the first tooth movements (up to a maximum of two) using the preference list given above. If you cannot use a palatal spring for any reason try a buccal spring etc. Screws are usually only required when the tooth to be retracted must also serve to retain the appliance.

Step 2

Plan posterior retention. Almost invariably this will involve Adams clasps on the first molars. If first molars have been extracted there will be problems which fall outside the scope of this book.

Step 3

Plan anterior retention. Here there is considerable room for flexibility (Adams clasps, short bows, long bows, Southend clasp). Try to engage a tooth as far labially as possible. Try also to place the retainer so as to permit desirable spontaneous movements to take place without interference. For example, there is no reason why an upper central and adjacent lateral should be clasped rather than the two central incisors.

Step 4

Outline the baseplate and add any bite planes required.

Step 5

Plan the anchorage. If in doubt add molar tubes to the bridges of the molar clasps so that the anchorage can be reinforced with headgear later if necessary.

Step 6

Improvements: ask yourself whether there is any way in which the appliance can be modified to allow the subsequent tooth movements in your plan to be carried out using the same appliance. Can further springs be incorporated at this stage to facilitate this? Does the design lend itself to modification at the chairside for example, by soldering or coldcuring in further active elements?

RETENTION

Before treatment is finally embarked upon a retention regime must be determined. This is because it affects the overall treatment time during which the patient will need to wear appliances.

No retention

Where the tooth alignment has been achieved by spontaneous improvement it is hardly likely to relapse. Such changes include the reduction of an overjet following the cessation of a digit-sucking habit and the spontaneous lower arch alignment which may follow first premolar extractions. Little if any retention will be needed for those tooth movements involving single teeth displaced by local factors, which have been aligned to positions which are obviously stable for adjacent teeth. Such instances are almost always confined to teeth in crossbite (which are also mechanically retained by the occlusion at the end of treatment) and permanent teeth which have been temporarily displaced by a retained precursor.

Standard retention period

Six months is usually regarded as the normal period of retention. This is because there is evidence to suggest that this is the time necessary for the principal fibres of the periodontal membrane to adapt to the tooth's new position. Some use this period for full-time retention and then discard the appliance but most favour a period of nights only retention. This allows any tendency to relapse to become apparent (through the appliance becoming slightly tight to insert) and enables the patient to dispense with daytime wear without any disadvantage provided the occlusion is regularly checked against post-treatment records. The authors' standard regime is 3 months' full-time wear and 3 months' nights only wear.

Long-term retention

This is needed for all rotations and for median diastemata. Permanent retention may have to be considered in some of these cases and is always necessary where orthodontic treatment has been carried out to re-align periodontally involved teeth. In such cases patients must be warned of this necessity at the treatment planning stage.

SECTION TWO

Pretreatment records

Turn to the inner front cover and carry out an examination of the following cases using this as a guide. We suggest you undertake no more than one or two at any occasion. Write down your findings and check these against the assessment provided in Section Three.

Note that in some cases the dates of the models and radiographs do not match.

Cases key

JB 10 years 3 months

NAME SEX
J.B. FEMALE

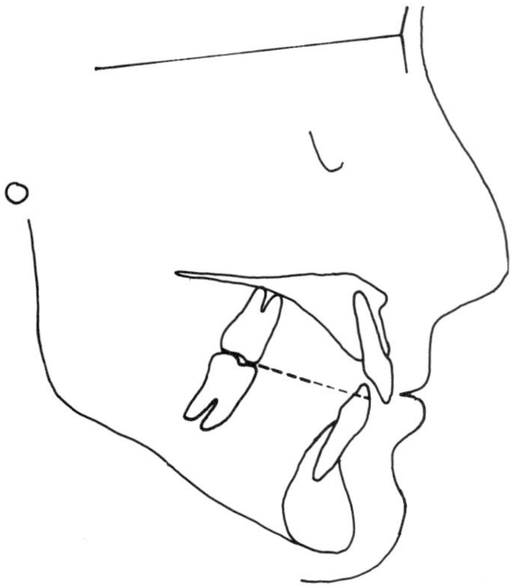

SKELETAL

SNA	°	79.0
SNB	°	75.5
ANB	°	3.0
SN/MxP	°	12.5
MxP/MnP	°	24.0
LAFH	mm	59.0
UAFH	mm	58.0
LAFH/TAFH	%	50.5
LPFH	mm	38.5
UPFH	mm	49.0
PFH	mm	74.0
Wits	mm	-1.5

TEETH

Overjet	mm	5.0
Overbite	mm	2.0
UI/MxP	°	111.0
LI/MnP	°	91.0
IIangle	°	134.5
LI-APo	mm	-0.5
LI-NPo	mm	-0.5

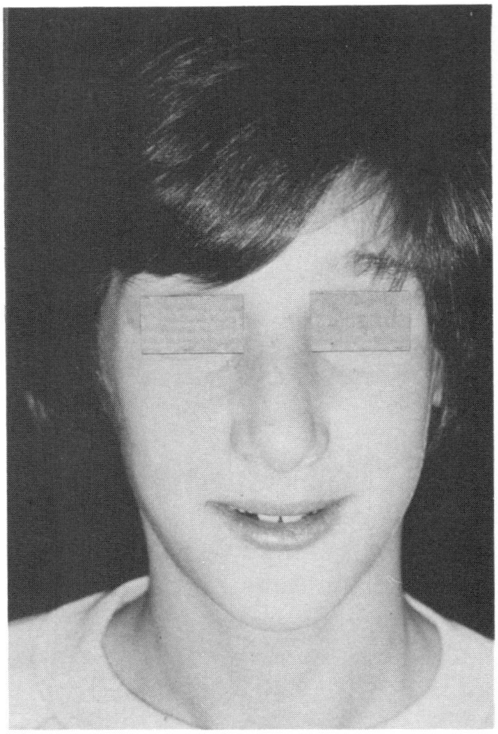

HISTORY

Reason for attendance

The patient was referred by her father, a university lecturer who was dentally qualified. Both parents were concerned about the late appearance and palatal displacement of the upper right canine. The patient herself was slightly concerned about crowding in the upper labial region.

Dental history

The patient had taken fluoride tablets from birth and had never had any dental treatment apart from removal of a mucous retention cyst carried out under local anaesthesia at 7 years.

Medical history

There was no relevant medical history.

SOFT TISSUES

The lips were mildly incompetent but habitually held together. The lower lip at rest just covered the upper incisal edges.

GENERAL CONDITION OF THE MOUTH

The patient had an excellent caries-free mouth with good oral hygiene and was dentally rather advanced for her age.

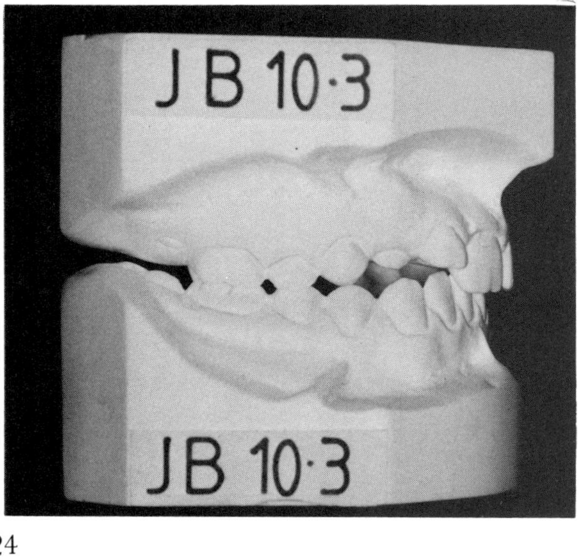

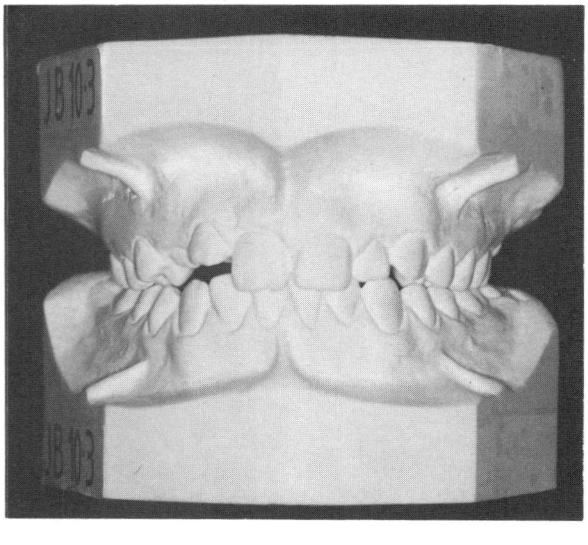

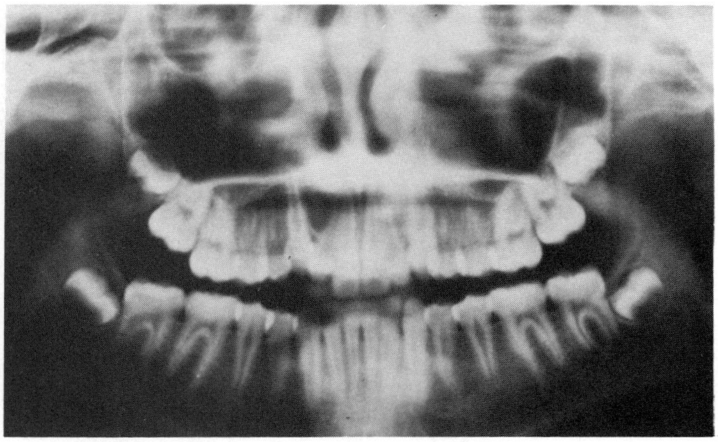

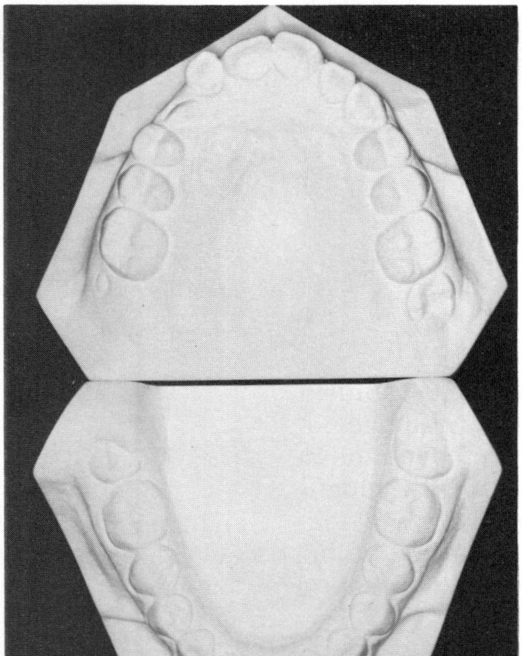

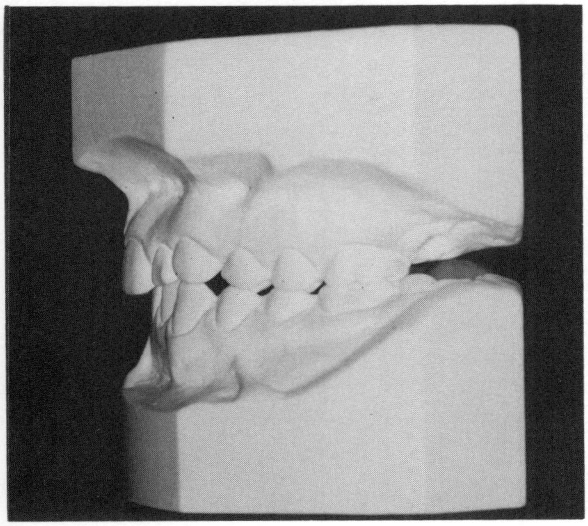

LB 23 years 3 months

NAME	SEX
L.B.	FEMALE

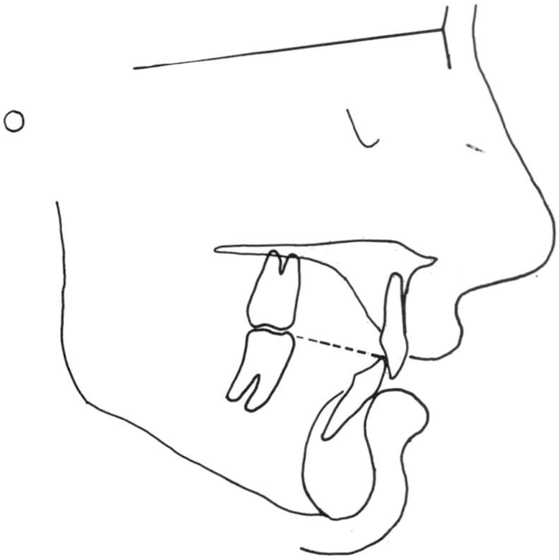

SKELETAL

SNA	°	76.0
SNB	°	72.0
ANB	°	4.5
SN/MxP	°	10.0
MxP/MnP	°	23.0
LAFH	mm	63.5
UAFH	mm	54.5
LAFH/TAFH	%	53.5
LPFH	mm	47.5
UPFH	mm	46.5
PFH	mm	78.5
Wits	mm	3.0

TEETH

Overjet	mm	2.5
Overbite	mm	4.5
UI/MxP	°	89.0
LI/MnP	°	103.5
IIangle	°	144.5
LI-APo	mm	-3.0
LI-NPo	mm	-1.5

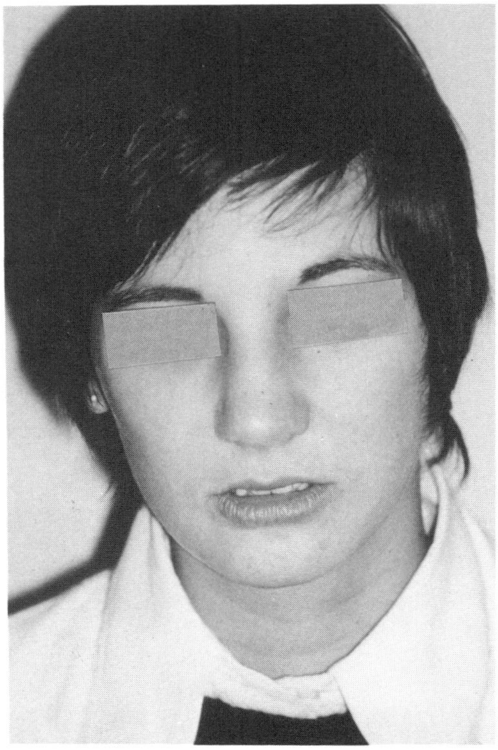

HISTORY

Reason for attendance

The patient was a third-year dental student who was quite happy with her appearance but had become concerned with the overeruption of the lower right second molar and the widening of the periodontal space of the lower right first molar which she judged to be due to the traumatic occlusion with the upper left second molar.

Dental history

She had received routine dental treatment for many years and had just completed having all past restorations replaced by a member of staff.

Medical history

There was no relevant medical history.

SOFT TISSUES

The lips were mildly incompetent but habitually held together. At rest the lower lip just covered the upper incisor tips.

GENERAL CONDITION OF THE MOUTH

The oral hygiene was good but the teeth were heavily restored.

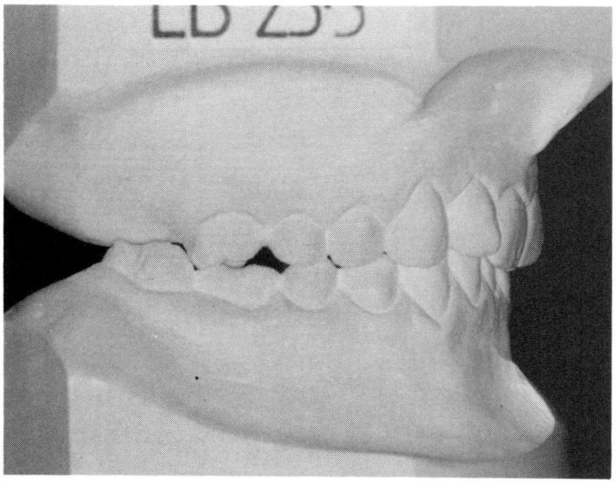

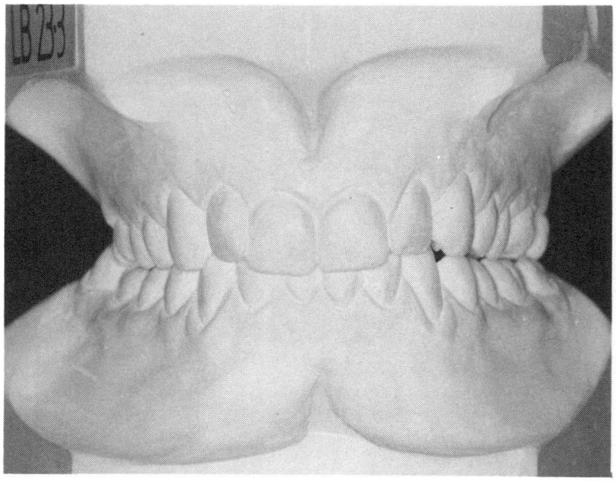

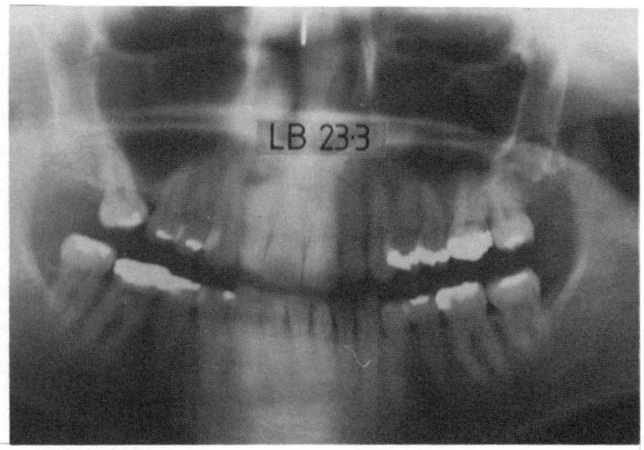
LB 23·3

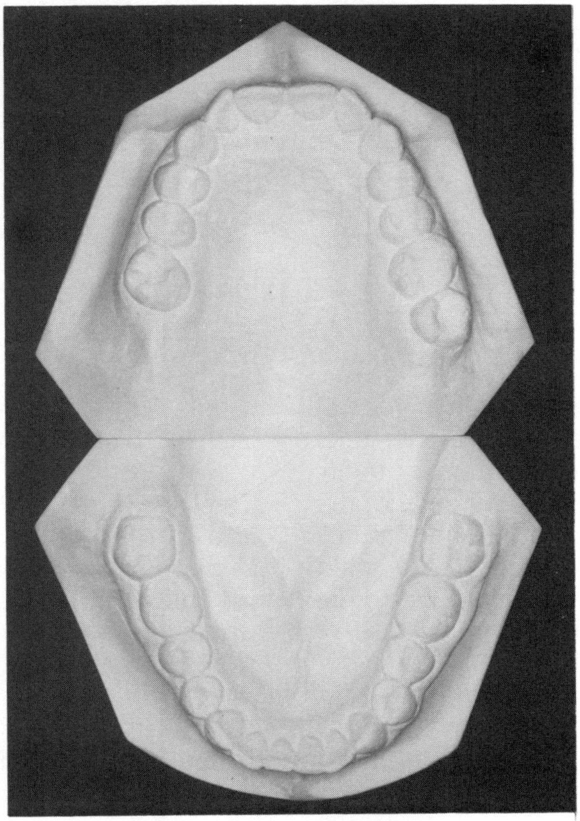

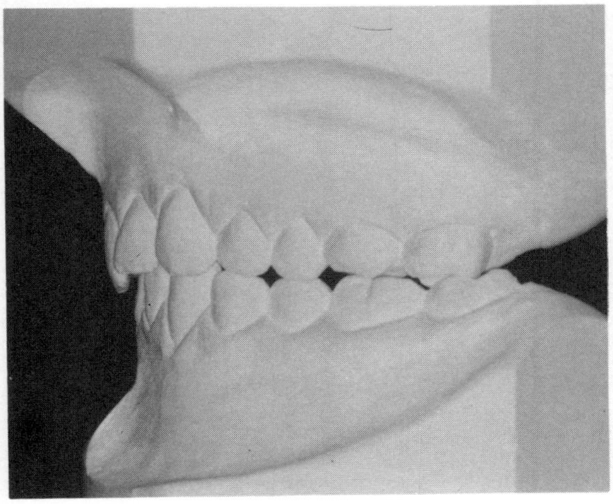

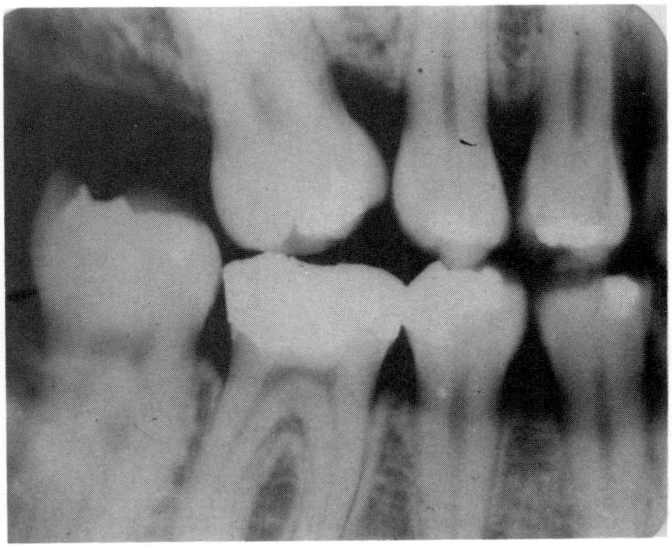

CB 10 years 1 month

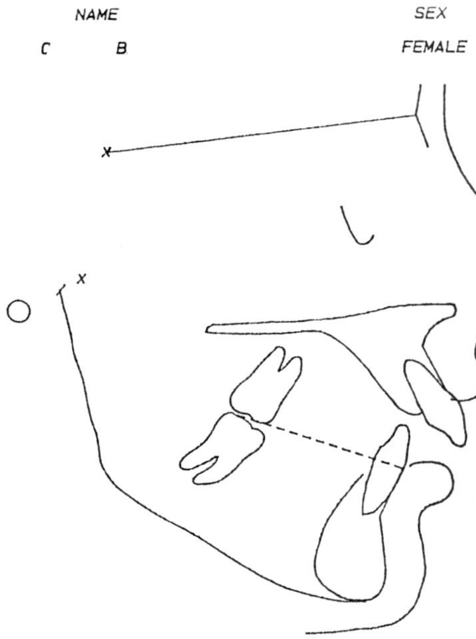

SKELETAL

SNA	°	84.5
SNB	°	78.0
ANB	°	6.5
SN/MxP	°	0.5
MxP/MnP	°	32.0
LAFH	mm	64.5
UAFH	mm	43.5
LAFH/TAFH	%	59.5
LPFH	mm	40.5
UPFH	mm	46.5
PFH	mm	76.5
Wits	mm	-3.5

TEETH

Overjet	mm	13.5
Overbite	mm	6.5
UI/MxP	°	115.5
LI/MnP	°	89.5
IIangle	°	123.0
LI-APo	mm	-1.0
LI-NPo	mm	2.0

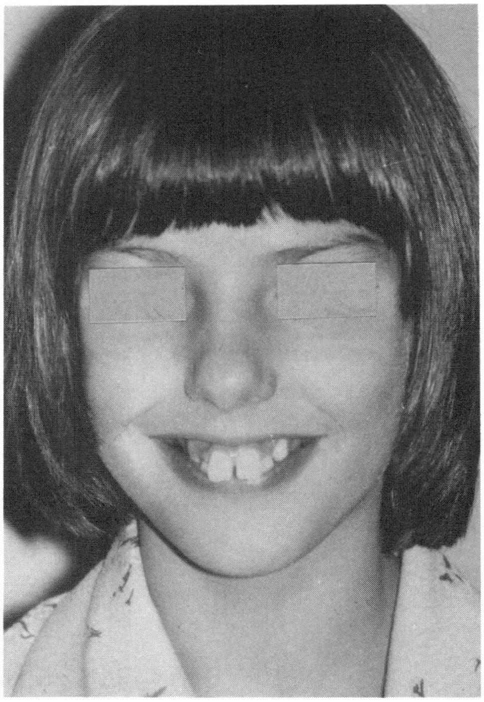

HISTORY

Reason for attendance

The patient had been referred by her general dental practitioner because, despite her age, both CB and her mother were keen for treatment to begin to correct the prominence of the upper incisors. Her mother had had multibanded fixed appliance treatment as a child and CB was well aware of what orthodontic treatment would probably entail.

Dental history

CB had been a regular attender with the family dental practitioner for several years.

Medical history

There was no relevant medical history.

SOFT TISSUES

The lips were grossly incompetent and habitually apart. At rest the lower lip lay just behind the upper incisor tips whilst the upper lip line was level with the gingival margins of the upper incisors. There was no history of a digit-sucking habit.

GENERAL CONDITION OF THE MOUTH

The oral hygiene was good and the caries rate low.

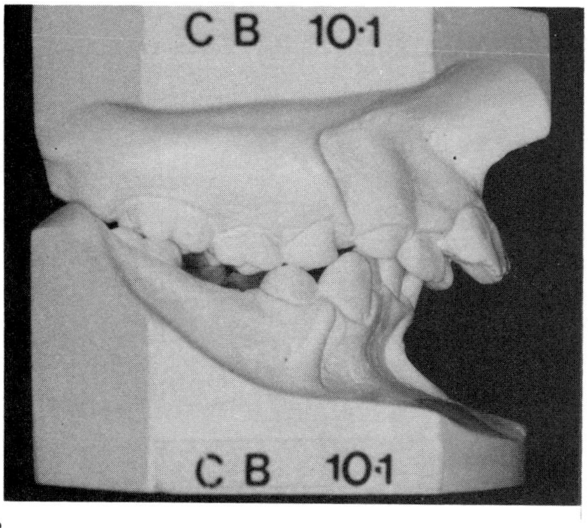

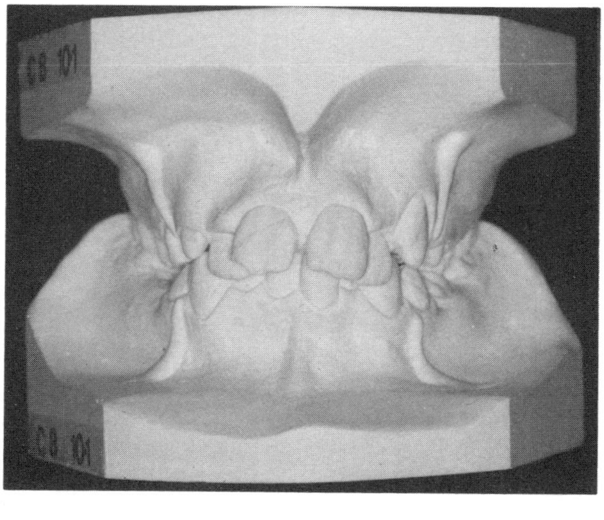

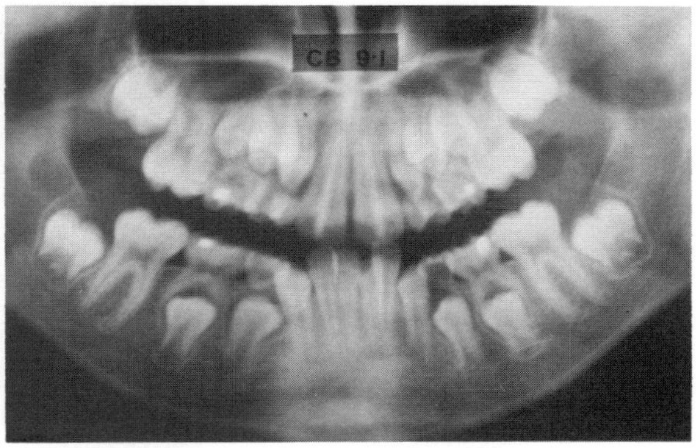
CB 9·1

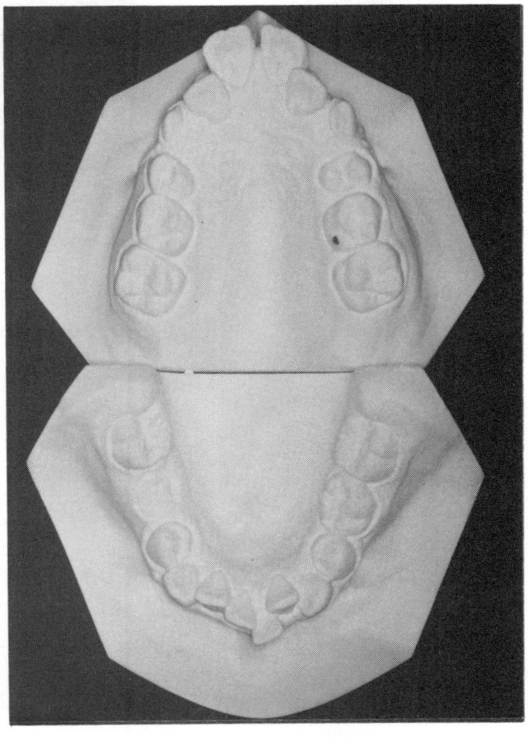

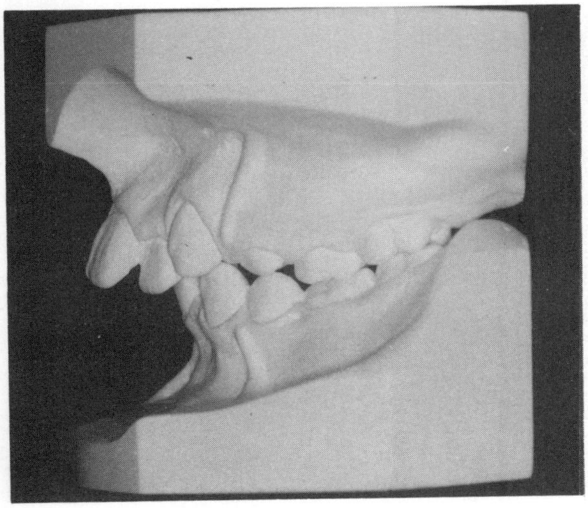

AT 13 years 2 months

NAME A.T.

SEX FEMALE

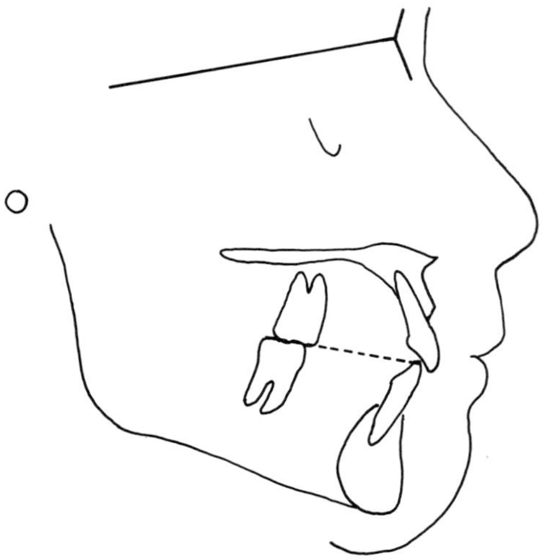

SKELETAL		
SNA	°	87.0
SNB	°	81.5
ANB	°	5.5
SN/MxP	°	10.0
MxP/MnP	°	18.0
LAFH	mm	59.5
UAFH	mm	50.5
LAFH/TAFH	%	54.0
LPFH	mm	46.0
UPFH	mm	46.5
PFH	mm	76.0
Wits	mm	−2.0
TEETH		
Overjet	mm	4.0
Overbite	mm	2.5
UI/MxP	°	112.5
LI/MnP	°	102.0
IIangle	°	128.0
LI-APo	mm	2.0
LI-NPo	mm	5.0

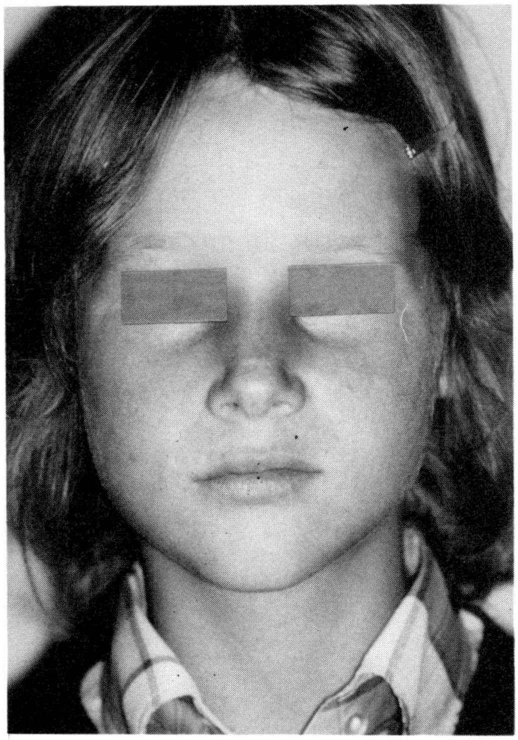

HISTORY

Reason for attendance

The patient was referred by her general dental practitioner for treatment of her lower incisor crowding, about which she was not greatly concerned.

Dental history

She had received regular dental treatment from the age of 6 years. She reported that the lower left second molar was giving her intermittent pain.

Medical history

There was no relevant medical history.

SOFT TISSUES

The lips were competent.

GENERAL CONDITION OF THE MOUTH

The oral hygiene was only fair.

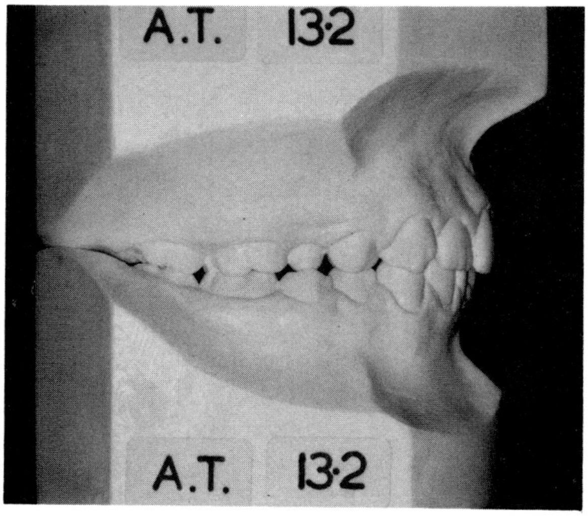

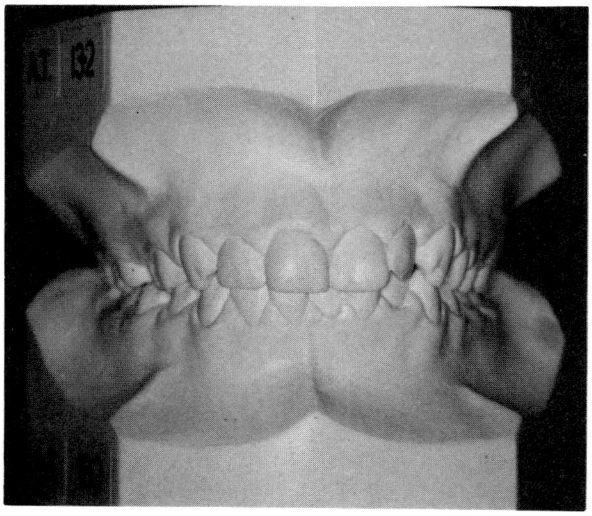

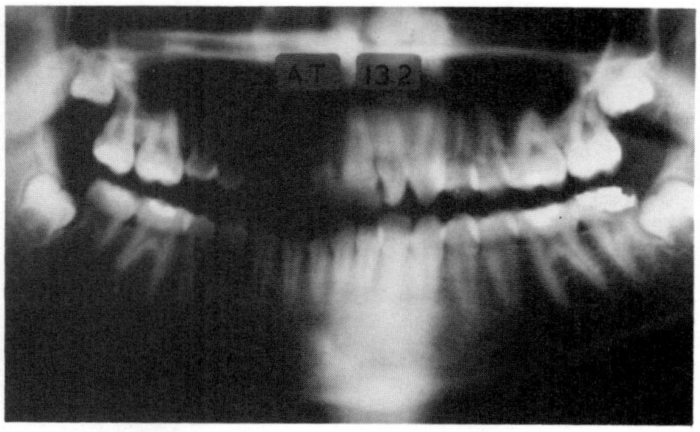
AT
13.2

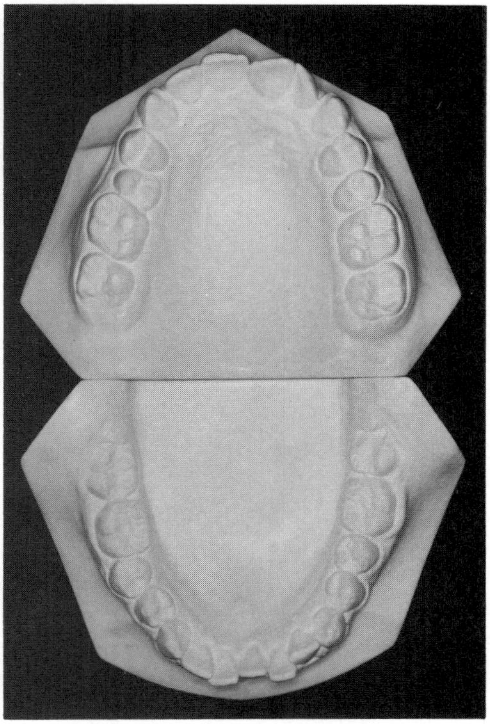

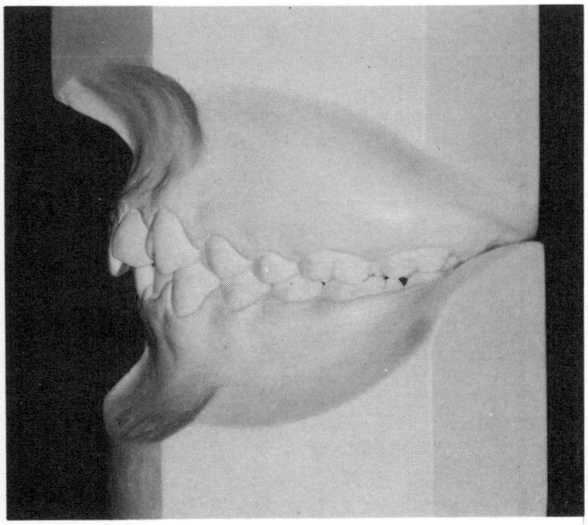

CW 11 years 11 months

NAME
C W

SEX
FEMALE

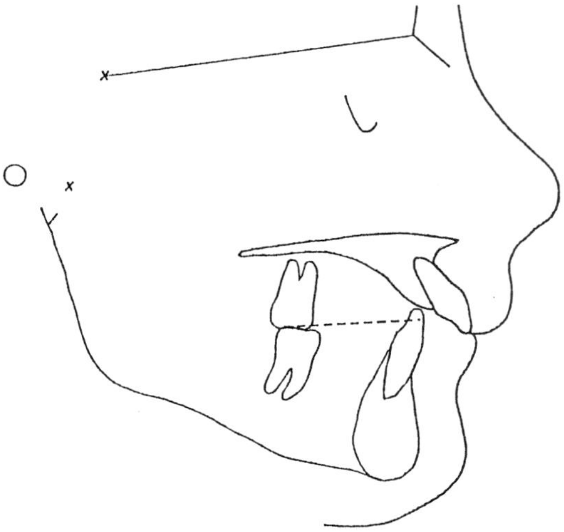

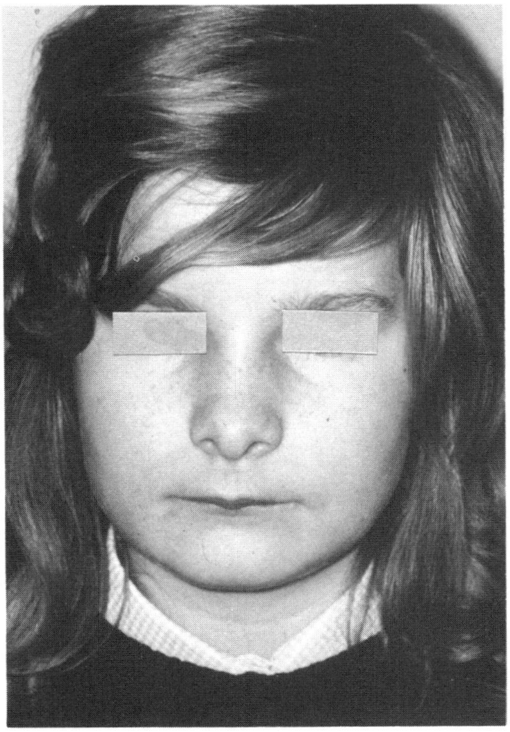

SKELETAL		
SNA	°	87.5
SNB	°	82.5
ANB	°	5.0
SN/MxP	°	3.5
MxP/MnP	°	24.5
LAFH	mm	54.0
UAFH	mm	48.5
LAFH/TAFH	%	52.5
LPFH	mm	41.0
UPFH	mm	52.5
PFH	mm	71.0
Wits	mm	6.0

TEETH		
Overjet	mm	11.0
Overbite	mm	6.0
UI/MxP	°	120.0
LI/MnP	°	90.5
IIangle	°	124.5
LI-APo	mm	−2.0
LI-NPo	mm	0.5

HISTORY

Reason for attendance

The family had recently moved to the area. The patient and her mother were concerned about soreness to the gum behind the upper central incisors.

Dental history

The family were regular dental attenders. CW had her upper deciduous central incisors avulsed at age 18 months.

Medical history

There was no relevant medical history.

Social history

The family live 12 miles away and have a car, although the patient is quite badly travel-sick.

SOFT TISSUES

The lips were mildly competent, habitually held together with the upper incisors trapped between them.

GENERAL CONDITION OF THE MOUTH

The oral hygiene was good.

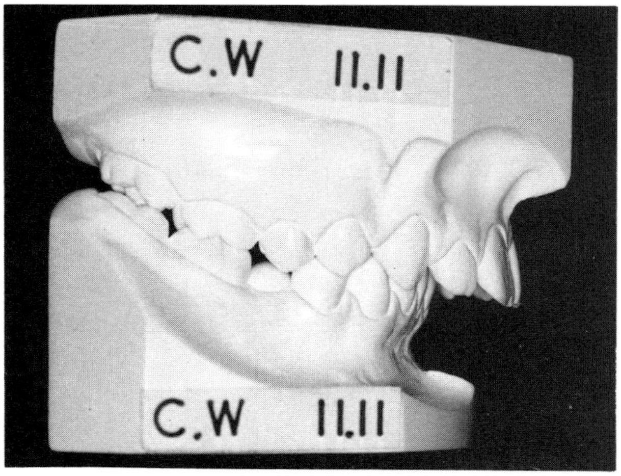

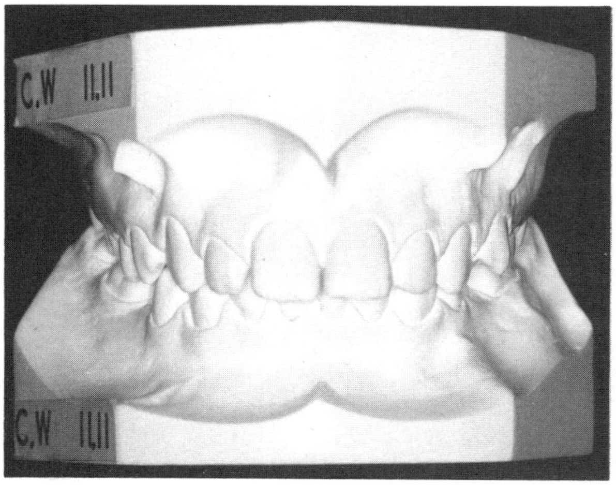

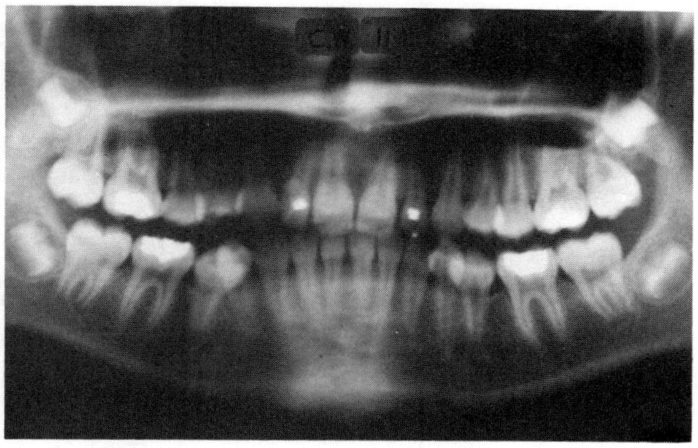

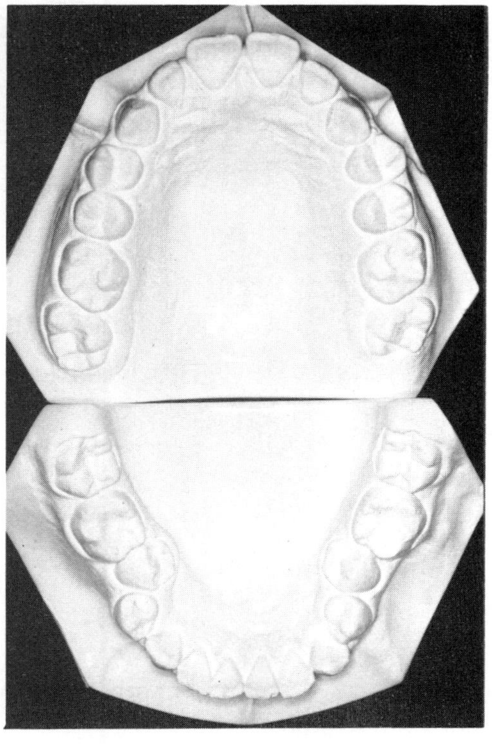

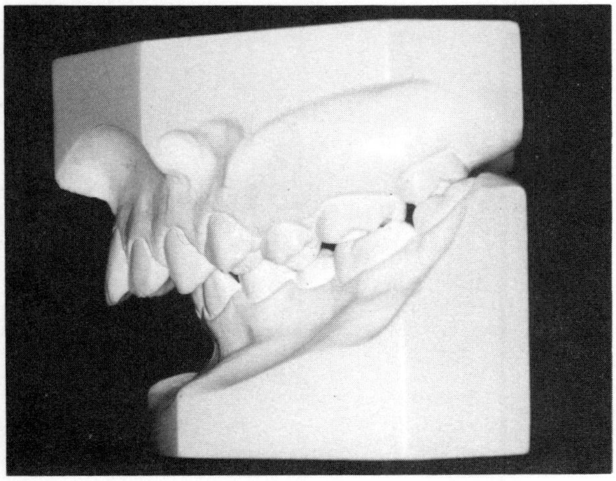

RP 9 years 9 months

NAME	SEX
R.P	FEMALE

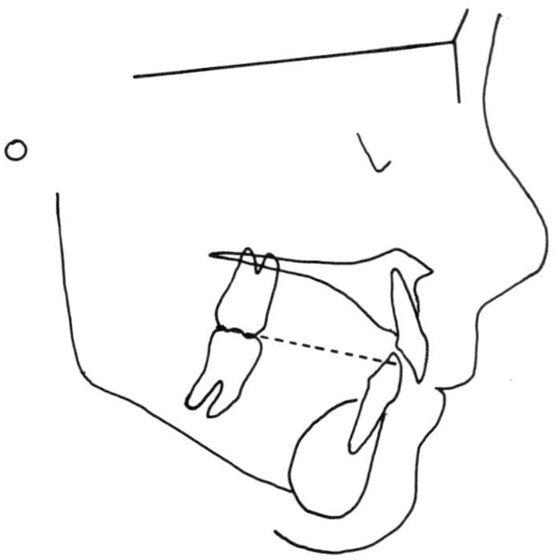

SKELETAL

SNA	°	74.0
SNB	°	73.0
ANB	°	1.0
SN/MxP	°	10.5
MxP/MnP	°	26.5
LAFH	mm	54.0
UAFH	mm	49.0
LAFH/TAFH	%	52.5
LPFH	mm	36.5
UPFH	mm	41.0
PFH	mm	64.0
Wits	mm	1.0

TEETH

Overjet	mm	5.0
Overbite	mm	5.5
UI/MxP	°	106.0
LI/MnP	°	87.5
IIangle	°	140.0
LI-APo	mm	0.0
LI-NPo	mm	0.5

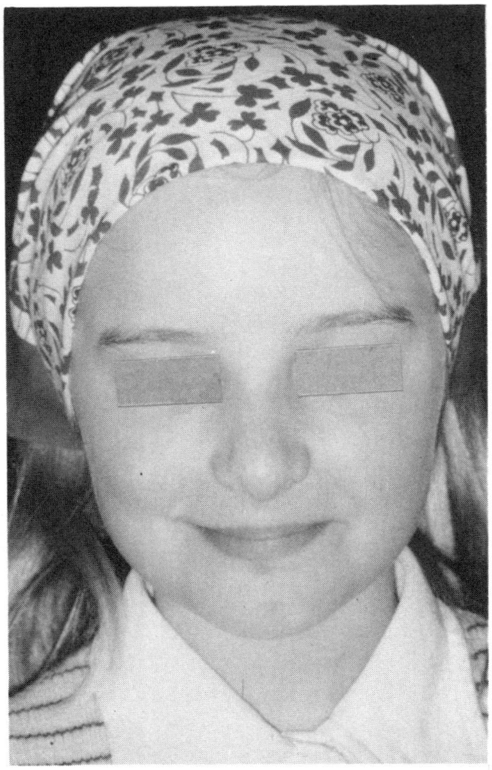

HISTORY

Reason for attendance

The patient had originally attended at 7 years of age, referred by her general dental practitioner because the patient's mother was concerned about very severe lower anterior crowding. The extraction of all four deciduous canines was advised at that time.

Dental history

The patient had received regular dental treatment from an early age.

Medical history

There was no relevant medical history.

SOFT TISSUES

The lips were competent and there was an average lip line (the lower lip rested one-third of the way up the labial surface of the upper incisors).

GENERAL CONDITION OF THE MOUTH

The oral hygiene was good.

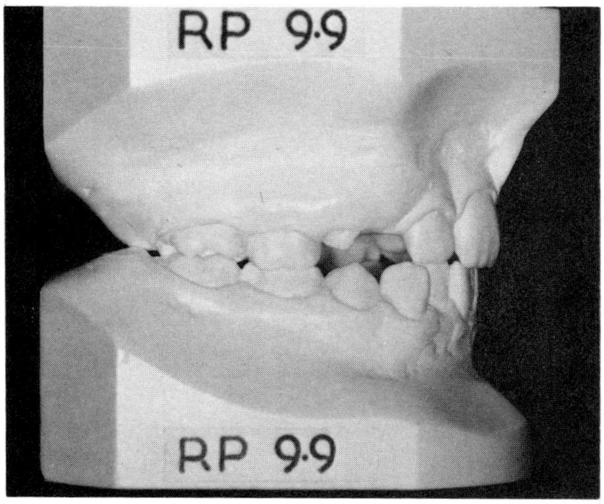

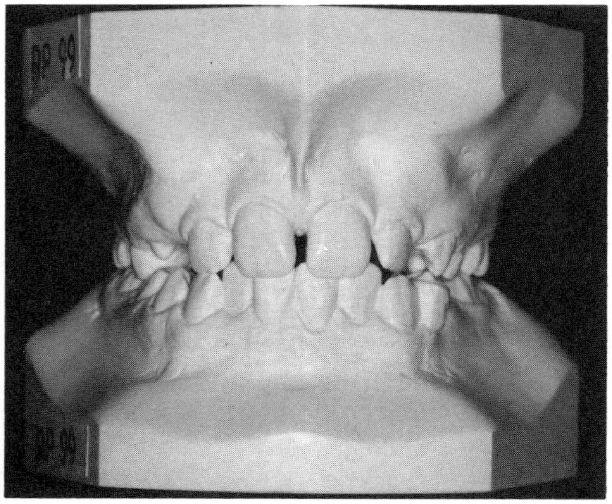

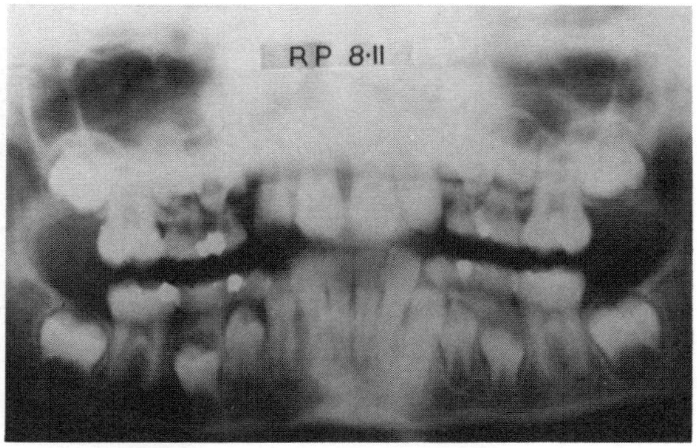
RP 8·11

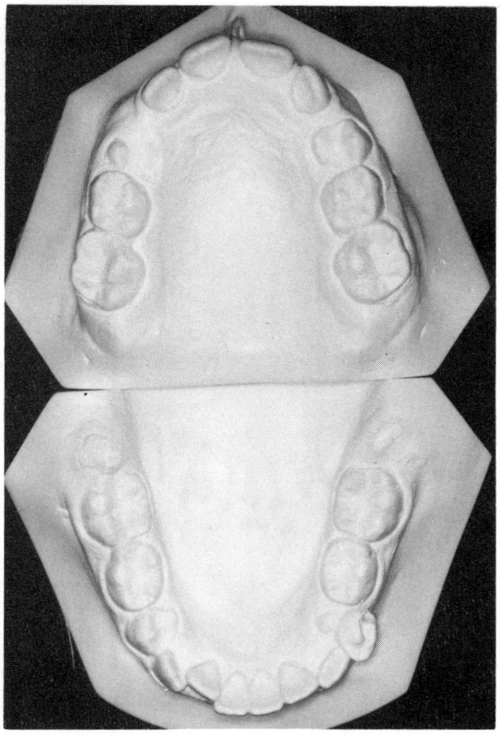

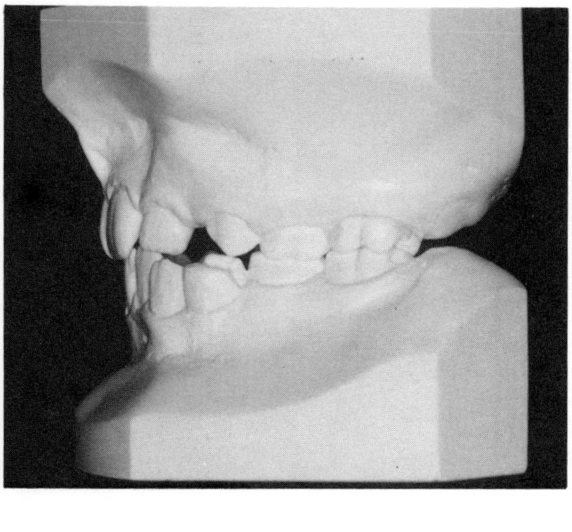

SD 11 years 4 months

NAME S.D.

SEX FEMALE

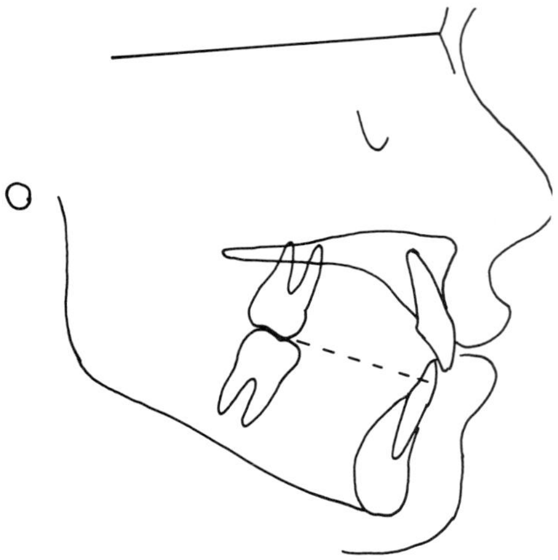

SKELETAL		
SNA	°	85.0
SNB	°	81.0
ANB	°	4.0
SN/MxP	°	0.5
MxP/MnP	°	29.5
LAFH	mm	61.0
UAFH	mm	47.0
LAFH/TAFH	%	56.5
LPFH	mm	40.5
UPFH	mm	51.5
PFH	mm	71.0
Wits	mm	−5.0
TEETH		
Overjet	mm	3.5
Overbite	mm	1.0
UI/MxP	°	103.5
LI/MnP	°	89.5
IIangle	°	138.0
LI-APo	mm	2.0
LI-NPo	mm	4.0

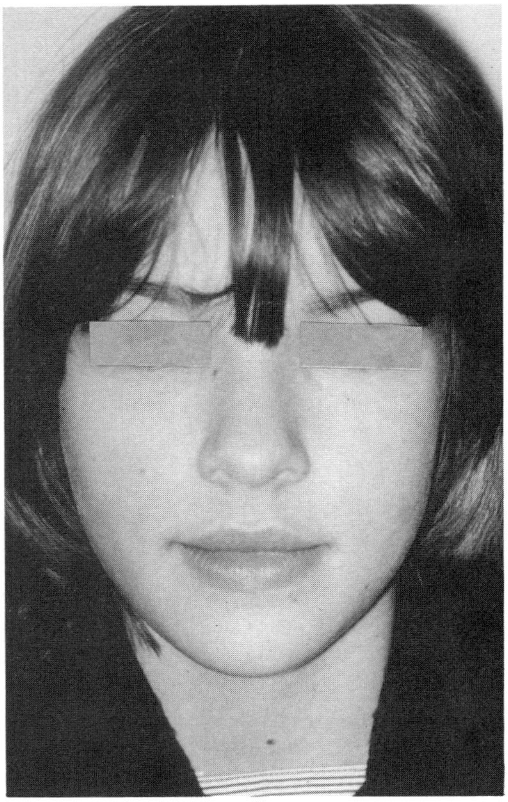

HISTORY

Reason for attendance

The patient was referred by her general dental practitioner who had noticed that the upper right lateral incisor had erupted into crossbite. The patient and parent were unconcerned.

Dental history

Although under the care of her family practitioner the patient was caries-free and at the time of first attending had never received any dental treatment apart from examinations.

Medical history

There was no relevant medical history.

SOFT TISSUES

The lips were competent.

GENERAL CONDITION OF THE MOUTH

The oral hygiene was excellent and the mouth was caries-free.

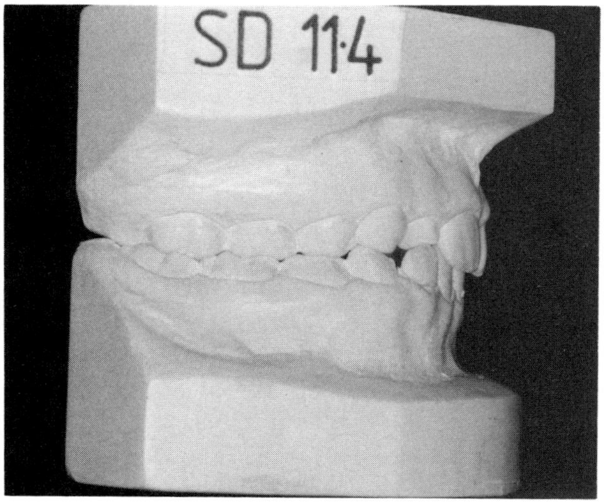

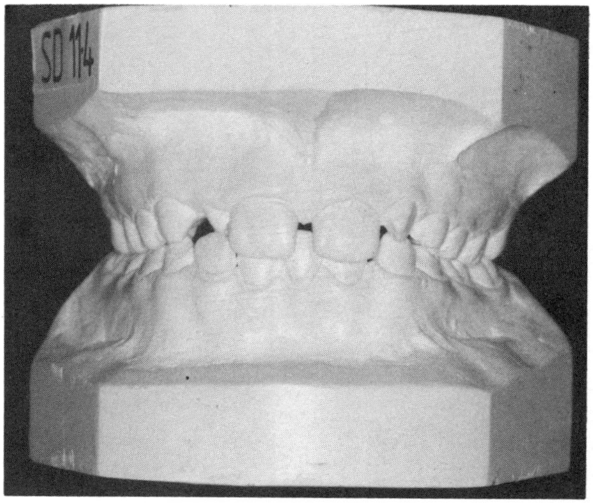

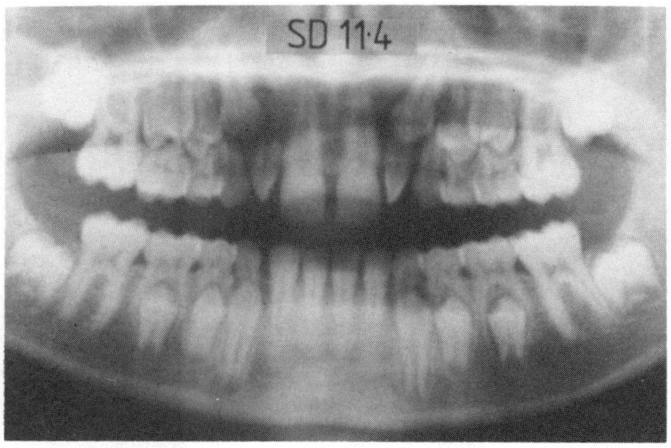
SD 11·4

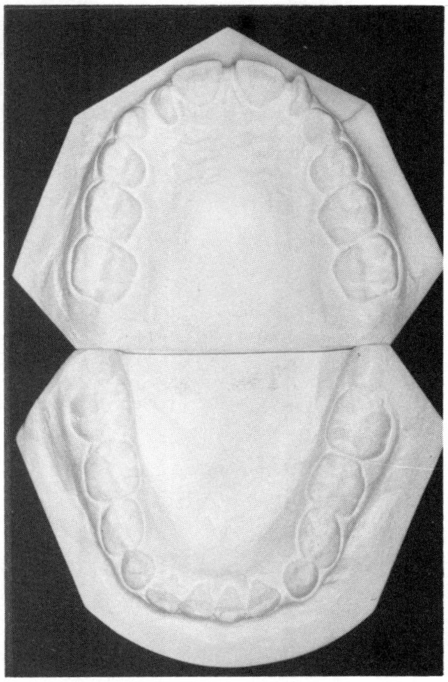

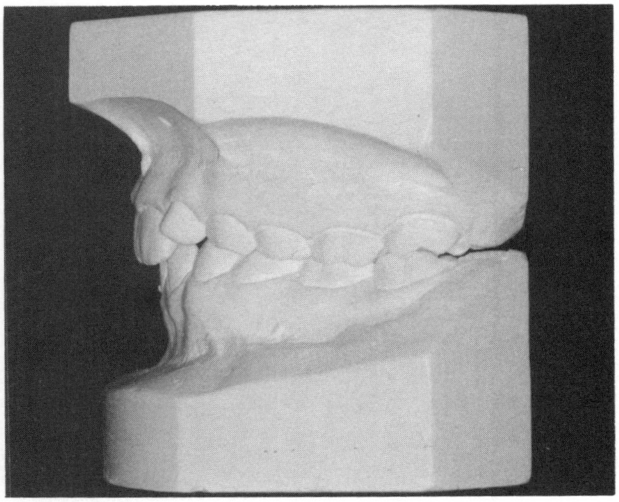

JK 11 years 7 months

NAME	SEX
J K	MALE

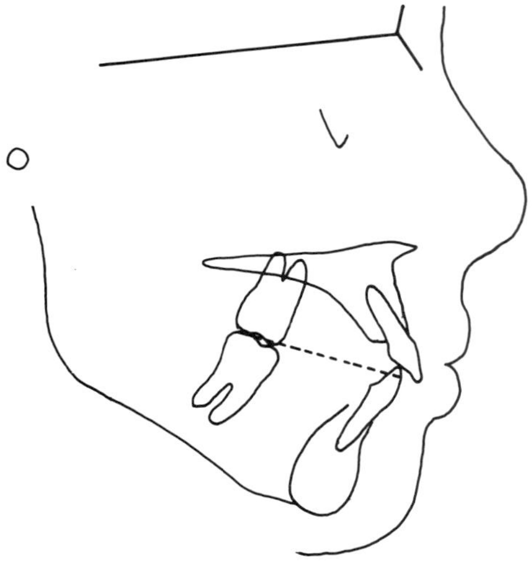

SKELETAL

SNA	°	83.0
SNB	°	79.0
ANB	°	4.0
SN/MxP	°	1.5
MxP/MnP	°	34.0
LAFH	mm	60.5
UAFH	mm	50.0
LAFH/TAFH	%	54.5
LPFH	mm	41.0
UPFH	mm	52.5
PFH	mm	70.5
Wits	mm	−4.0

TEETH

Overjet	mm	5.0
Overbite	mm	2.0
UI/MxP	°	112.0
LI/MnP	°	102.5
IIangle	°	111.5
LI-APo	mm	5.5
LI-NPo	mm	7.5

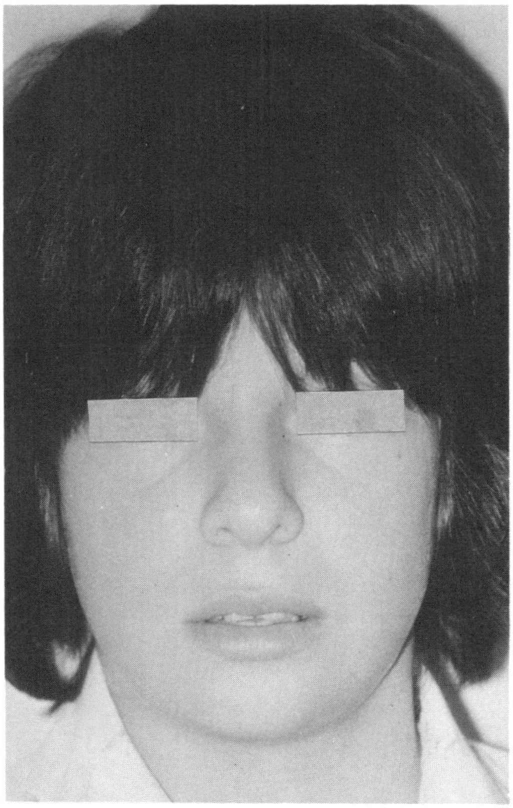

HISTORY

Reason for attendance

The patient had been referred by his general practitioner, a dental officer in the Community Dental Service. The boy was not unduly concerned about his malocclusion but accepted the idea of simple treatment.

Dental history

The patient had received routine dental treatment from the age of 5 years.

Medical history

There was no relevant medical history.

SOFT TISSUES

The lips were slightly incompetent but held together some of the time.

GENERAL CONDITION OF THE MOUTH

The oral hygiene was good.

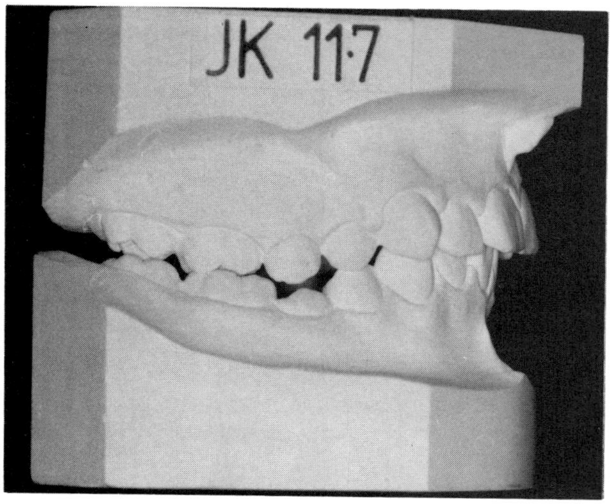

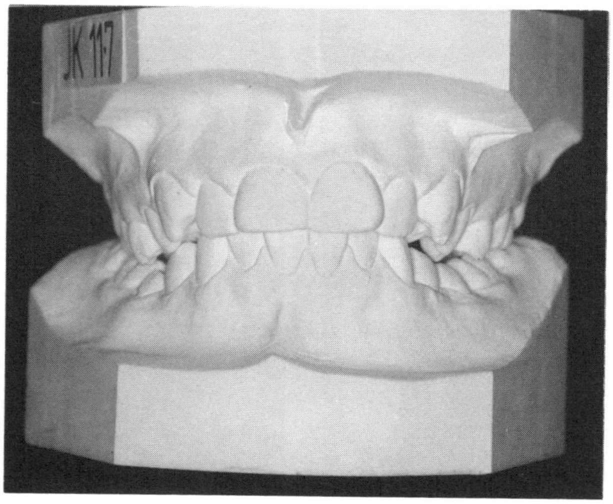

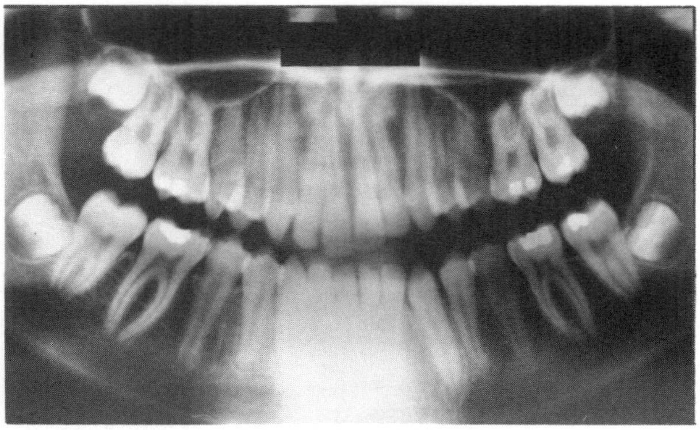

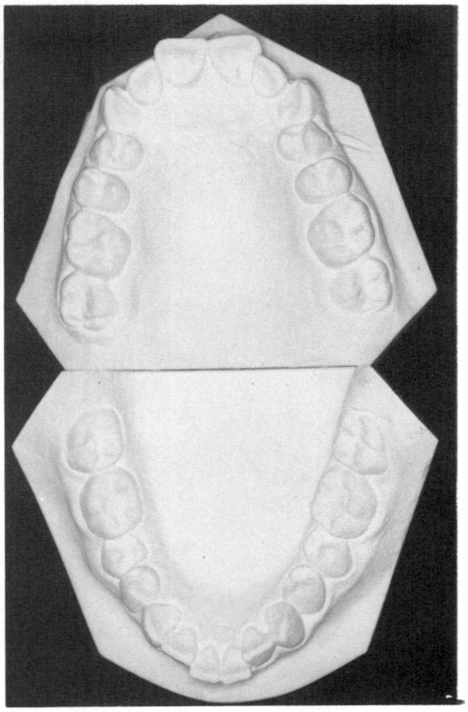

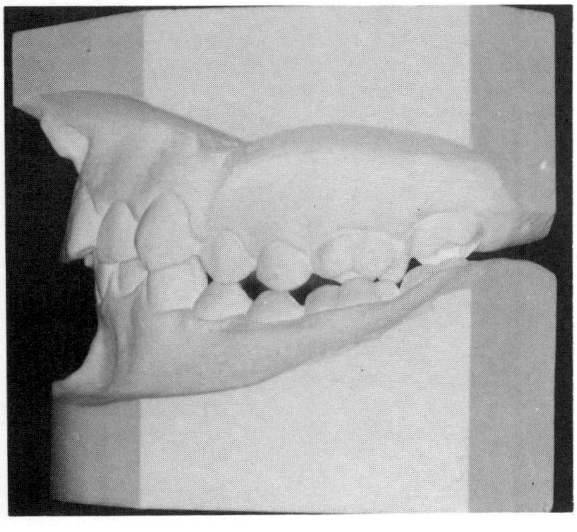

JA 10 years 5 months

NAME	SEX
J. A.	FEMALE

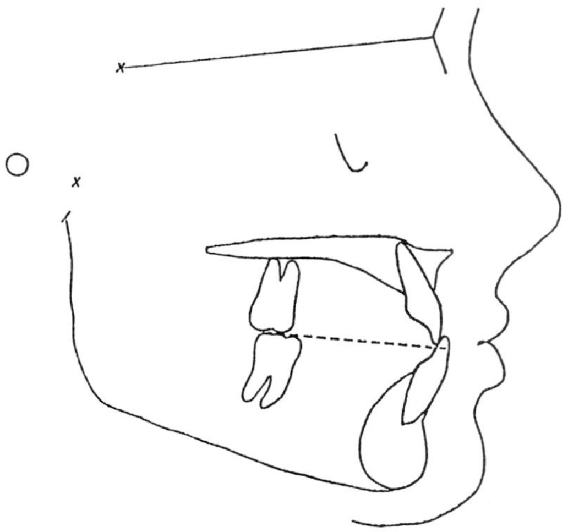

SKELETAL		
SNA	°	85.5
SNB	°	83.0
ANB	°	2.5
SN/MxP	°	6.0
MxP/MnP	°	17.0
LAFH	mm	54.5
UAFH	mm	49.0
LAFH/TAFH	%	52.5
LPFH	mm	42.0
UPFH	mm	46.0
PFH	mm	76.5
Wits	mm	0.0
TEETH		
Overjet	mm	-1.5
Overbite	mm	2.5
UI/MxP	°	114.0
LI/MnP	°	98.0
IIangle	°	131.0
LI-APo	mm	2.5
LI-NPo	mm	3.5

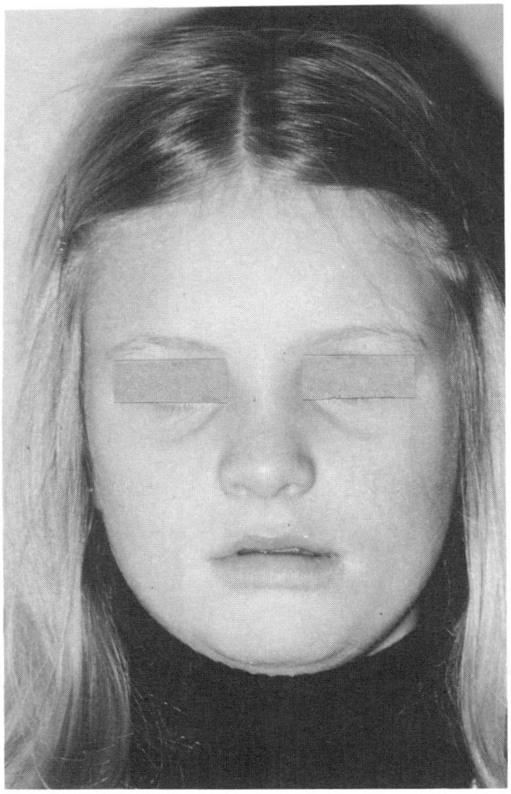

HISTORY

Reason for attendance

The patient's general practitioner was concerned about the developing Class III incisor relationship.

Dental history

The patient had received routine treatment from the family practitioner. This included extraction under local anaesthesia. There was a history of poor dietary control of fermentable carbohydrate but this had been corrected.

Medical history

There was no relevant medical history.

SOFT TISSUES

The lips were competent.

GENERAL CONDITION OF THE MOUTH

The oral hygiene was now good.

N.B.: It was not possible to detect a displacement on closure.

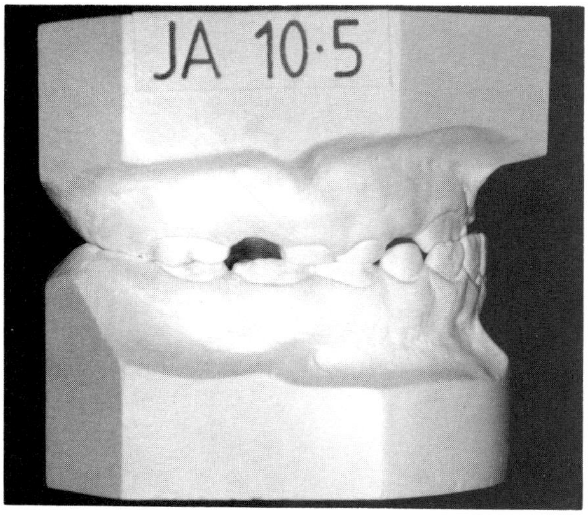

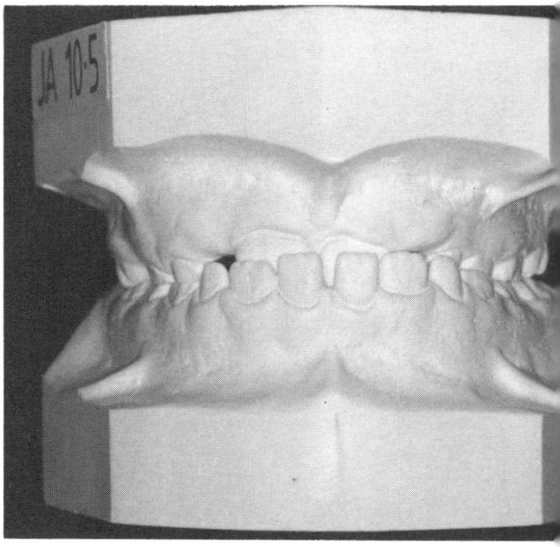

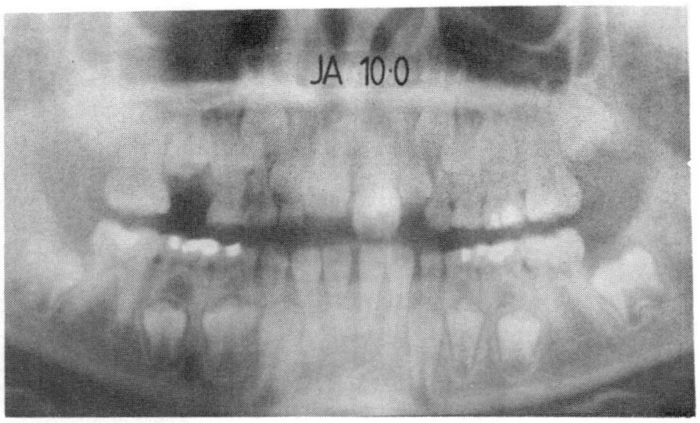
JA 10·0

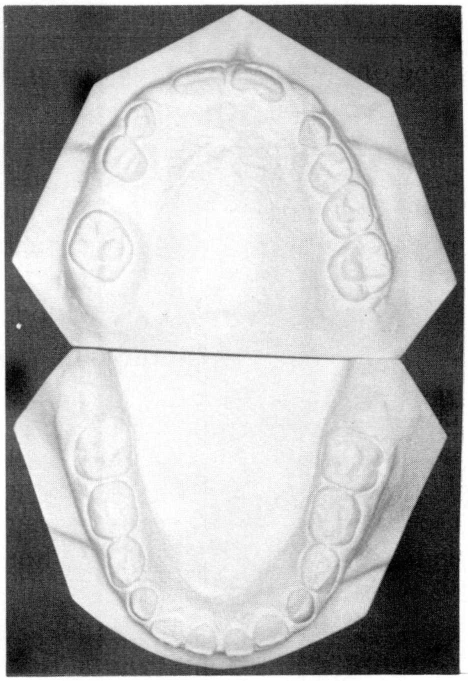

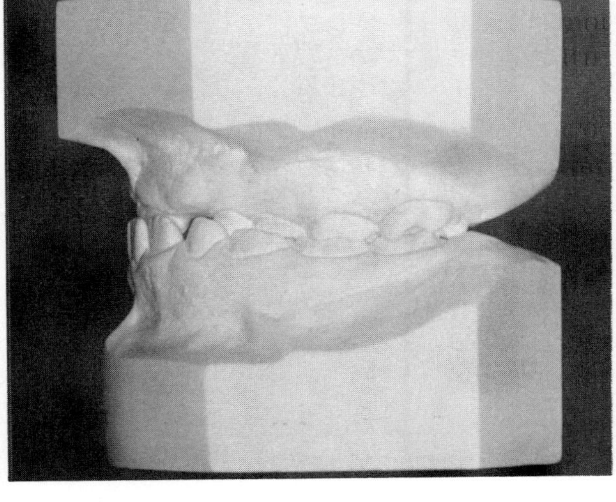

SN 11 years

NAME S.N.

SEX FEMALE

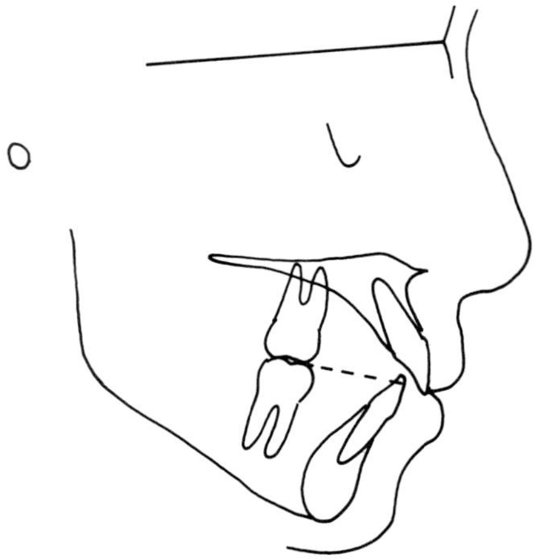

SKELETAL

SNA	°	75.0
SNB	°	74.0
ANB	°	1.5
SN/MxP	°	8.0
MxP/MnP	°	27.5
LAFH	mm	54.0
UAFH	mm	48.0
LAFH/TAFH	%	53.0
LPFH	mm	35.5
UPFH	mm	42.5
PFH	mm	67.5
Wits	mm	2.0

TEETH

Overjet	mm	5.0
Overbite	mm	1.5
UI/MxP	°	113.5
LI/MnP	°	99.5
IIangle	°	119.5
LI-APo	mm	4.5
LI-NPo	mm	5.0

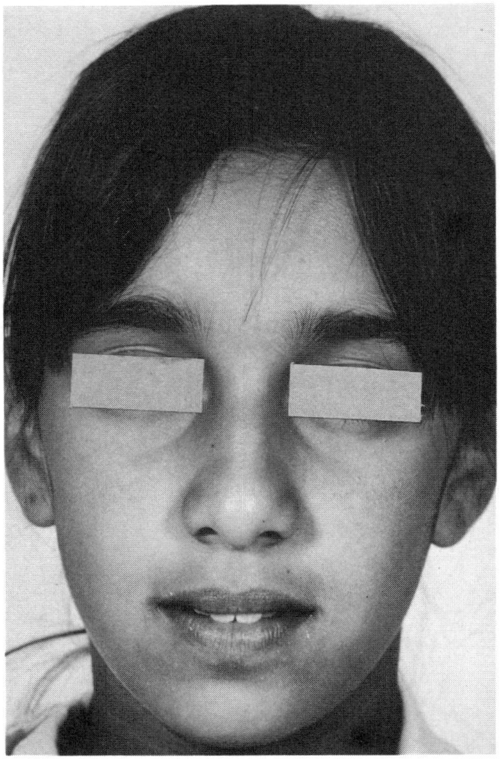

HISTORY

Reason for attendance

The father was a hospital consultant and had asked for an opinion as the family lived close to the unit.

Dental history

The patient was a regular attender for routine dental treatment.

Medical history

There was no relevant medical history.

SOFT TISSUES

The lips were competent but slightly everted in form.

GENERAL CONDITION OF THE MOUTH

The oral hygiene was only average.

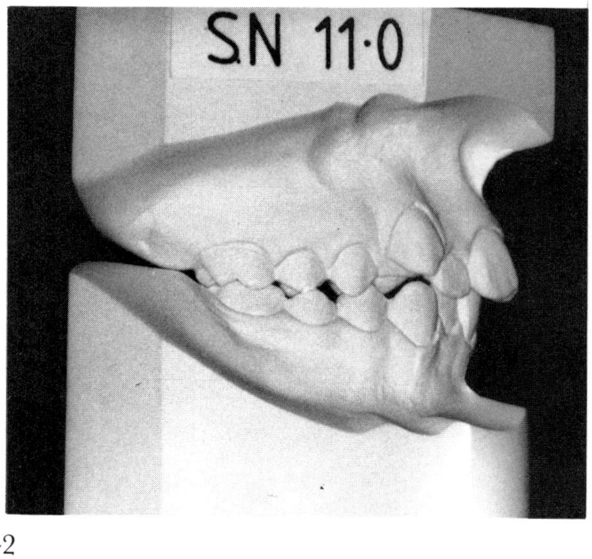

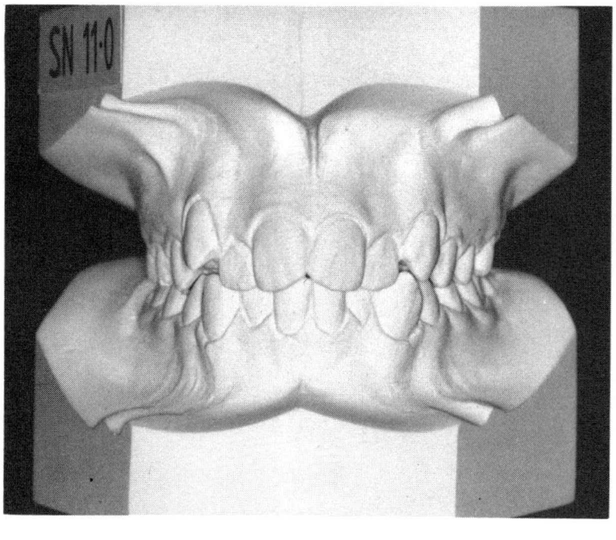

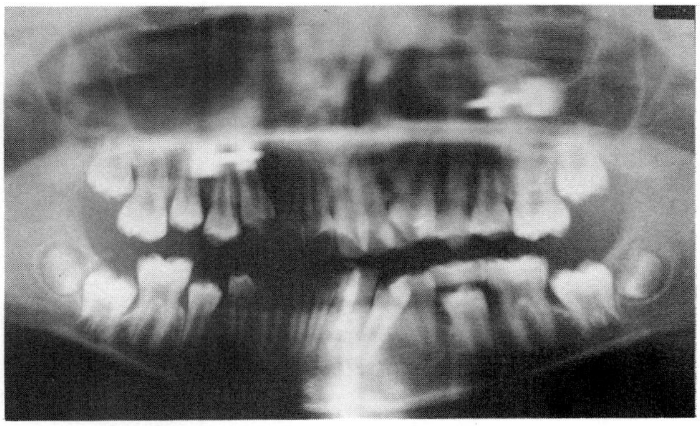

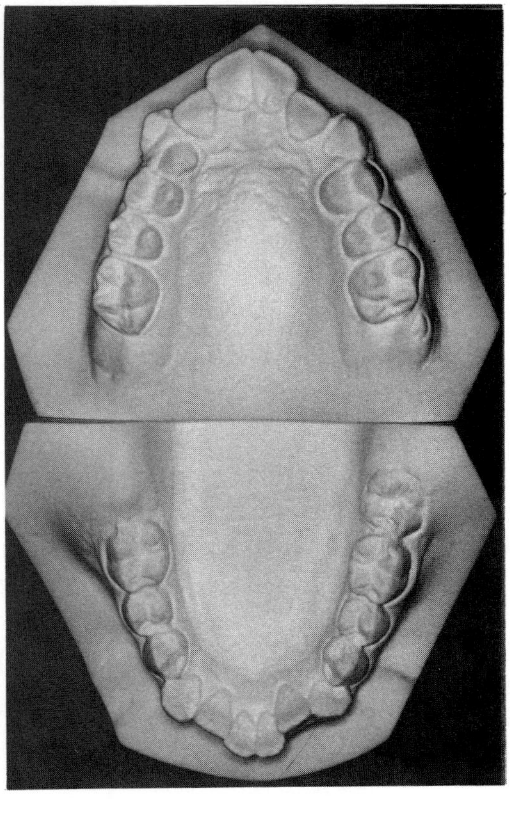

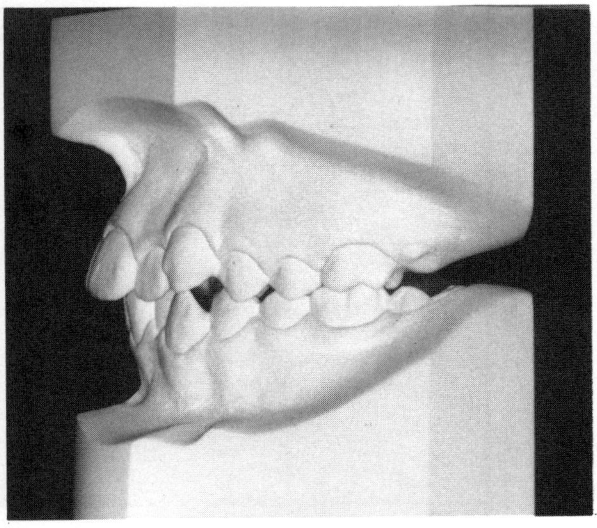

EH 13 years 11 months

NAME E.H.

SEX FEMALE

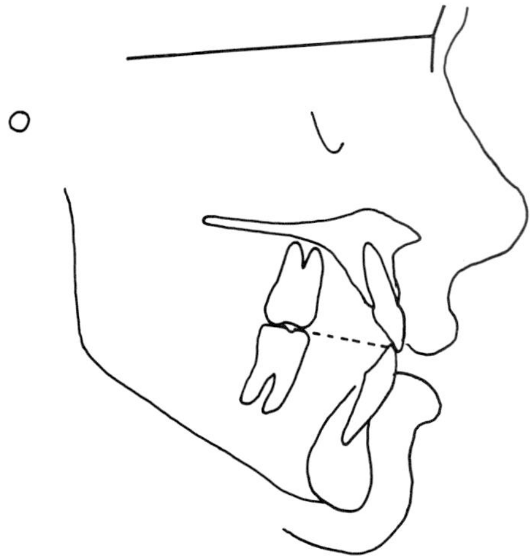

SKELETAL

SNA	°	75.5
SNB	°	76.5
ANB	°	-1.0
SN/MxP	°	9.5
MxP/MnP	°	25.0
LAFH	mm	62.0
UAFH	mm	45.5
LAFH/TAFH	%	57.5
LPFH	mm	40.0
UPFH	mm	39.5
PFH	mm	69.5
Wits	mm	-1.5

TEETH

Overjet	mm	1.5
Overbite	mm	1.0
UI/MxP	°	109.5
LI/MnP	°	88.5
IIangle	°	136.5
LI-APo	mm	1.0
LI-NPo	mm	-0.5

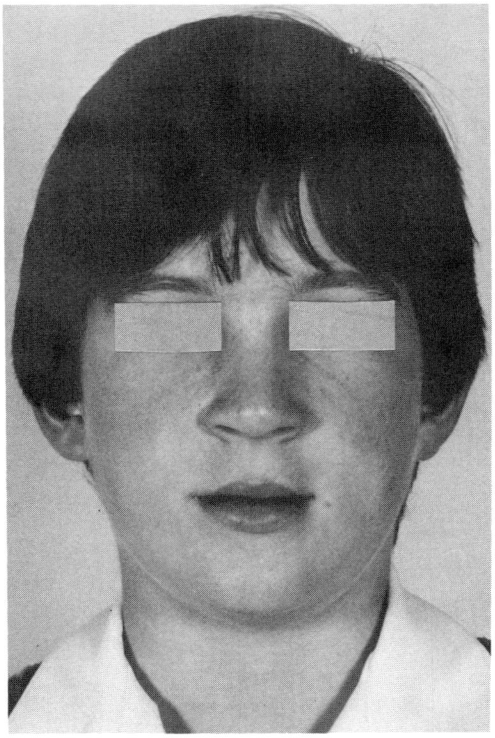

HISTORY

Reason for attendance

The patient had been referred because she and her mother were concerned about the appearance of the upper anterior teeth.

Dental history

The patient has been a regular dental attender with her general dental practitioner.

Medical history

There was no relevant medical history.

SOFT TISSUES

The lips were apart at rest but the upper lip covered the greater part of the upper incisors.

GENERAL CONDITION OF THE MOUTH

The oral hygiene was good.

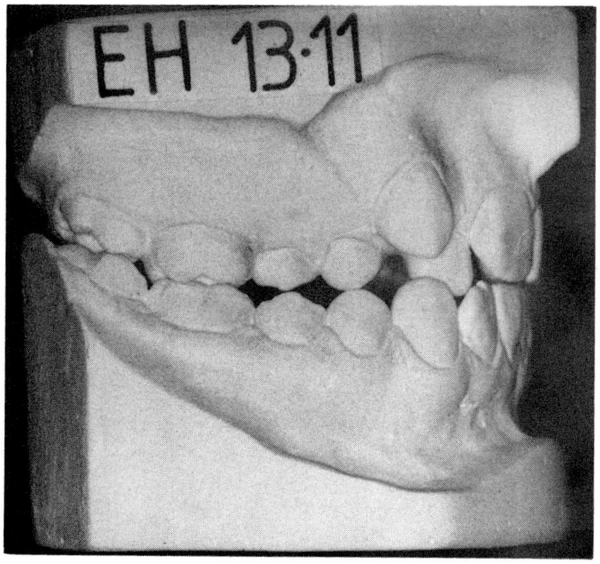

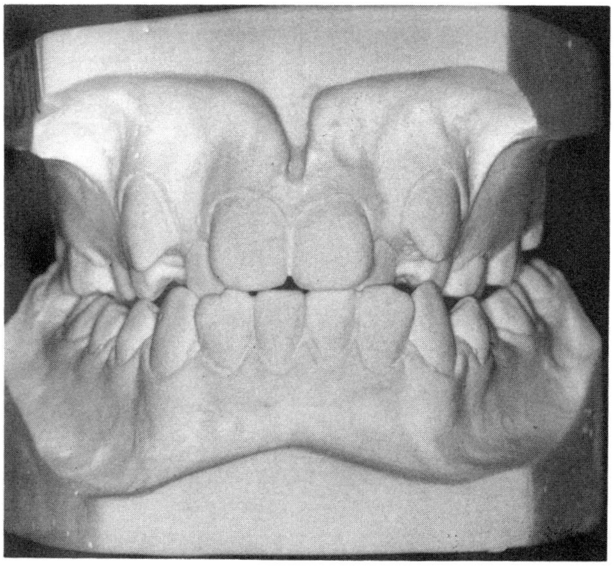

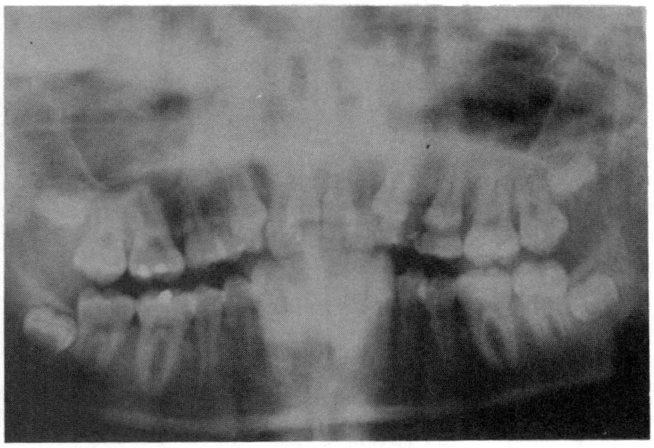

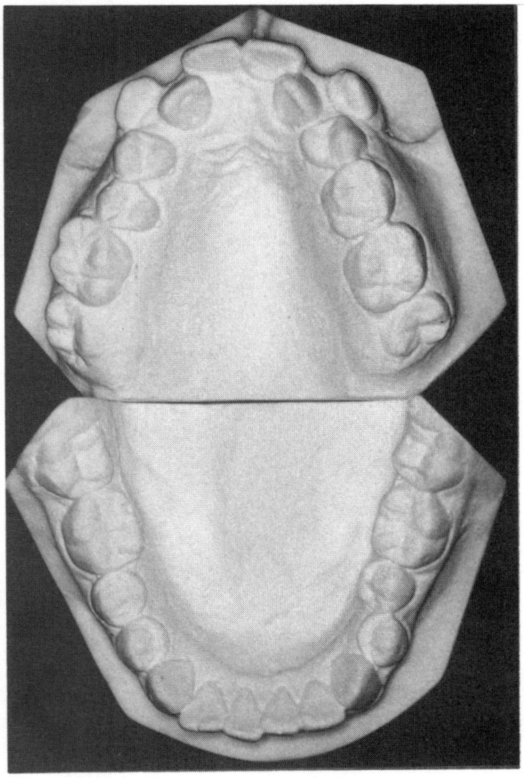

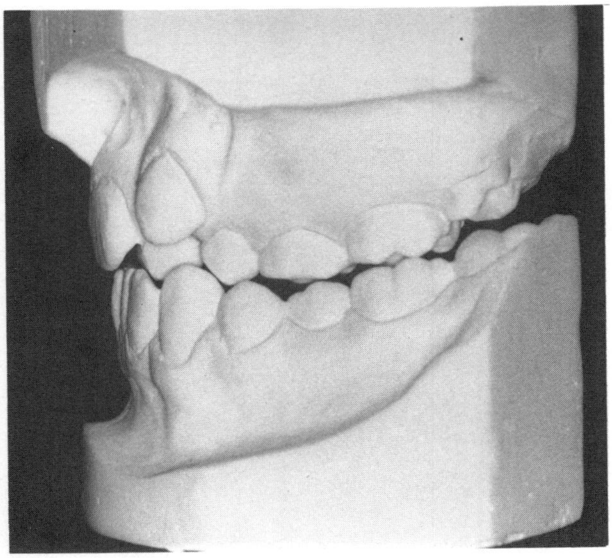

MB 12 years 10 months

NAME M.B.

SEX MALE

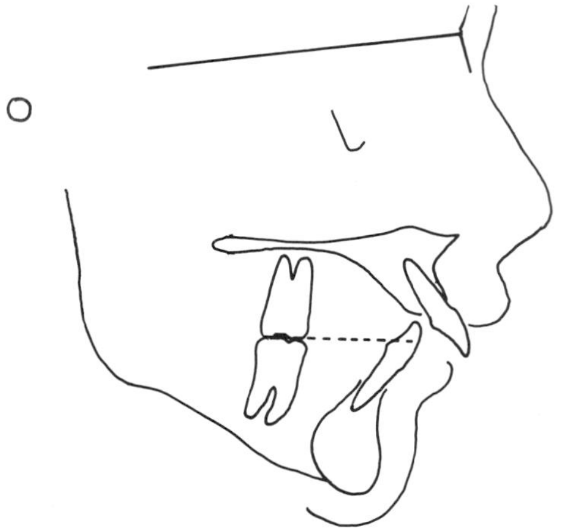

SKELETAL

SNA	°	77.0
SNB	°	71.0
ANB	°	6.0
SN/MxP	°	4.0
MxP/MnP	°	28.5
LAFH	mm	56.0
UAFH	mm	45.0
LAFH/TAFH	%	55.5
LPFH	mm	35.5
UPFH	mm	42.0
PFH	mm	67.5
Wits	mm	12.0

TEETH

Overjet	mm	10.5
Overbite	mm	6.5
UI/MxP	°	121.0
LI/MnP	°	104.5
IIangle	°	106.0
LI-APo	mm	0.0
LI-NPo	mm	2.5

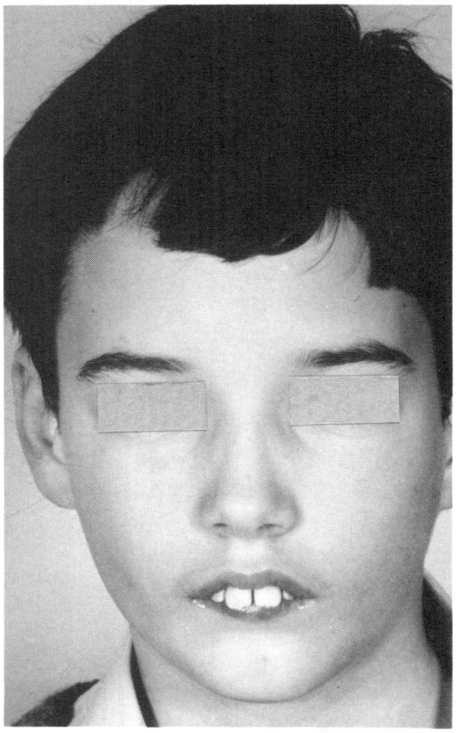

HISTORY

Reason for attendance

The patient had been referred by his practitioner for orthodontic advice. Both parent and patient were only slightly concerned about the malocclusion.

Dental history

The patient was a regular dental attender.

Medical history

There was no relevant medical history.

Social history

Unfortunately the family lived 32 miles from the unit and travel was difficult since the family had no car.

SOFT TISSUES

The lips were incompetent with the lower lip trapped behind the upper incisors.

GENERAL CONDITION OF THE MOUTH

The oral hygiene was only fair and there were extensive restorations in all four first permanent molars.

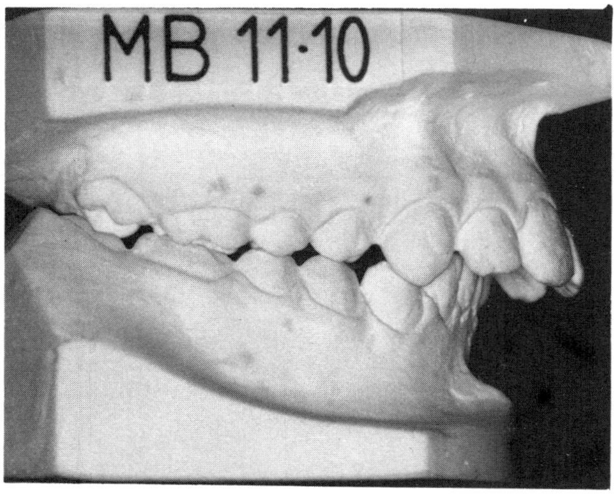

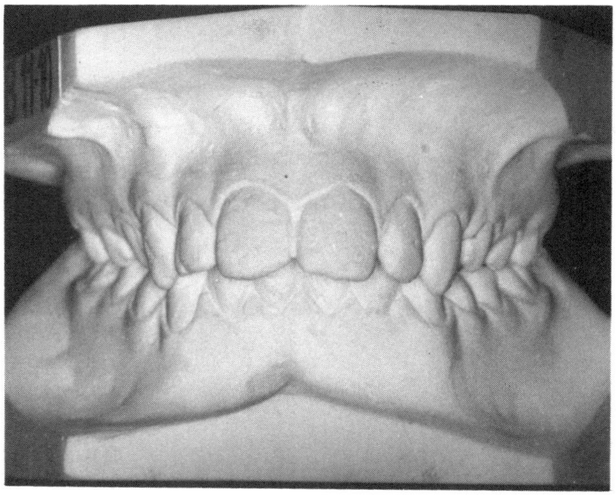

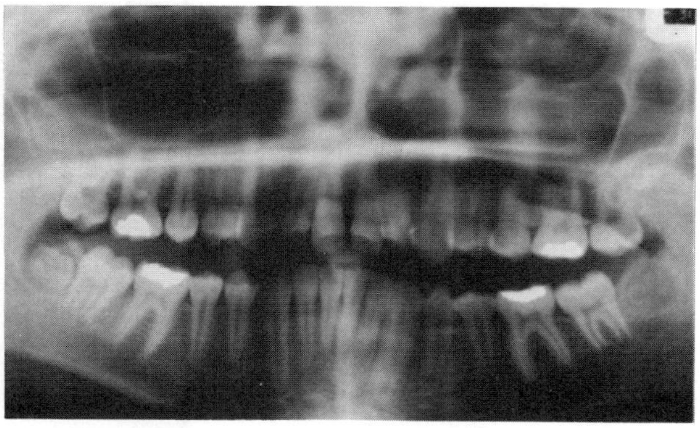

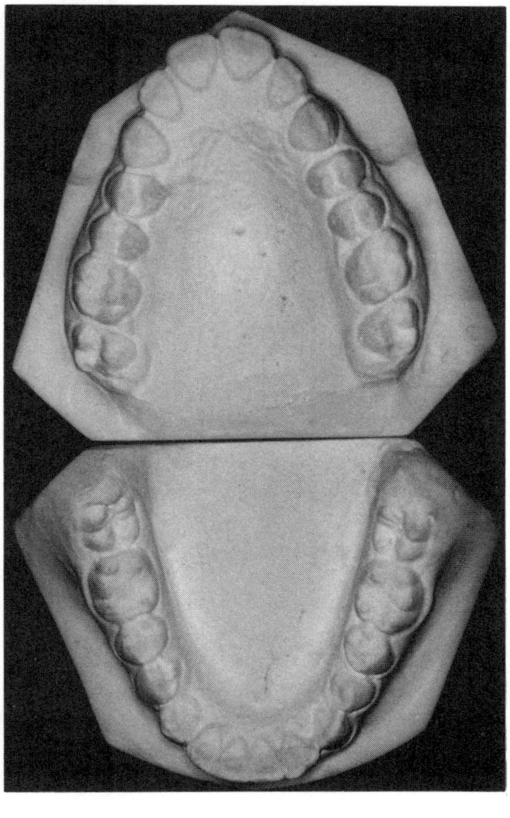

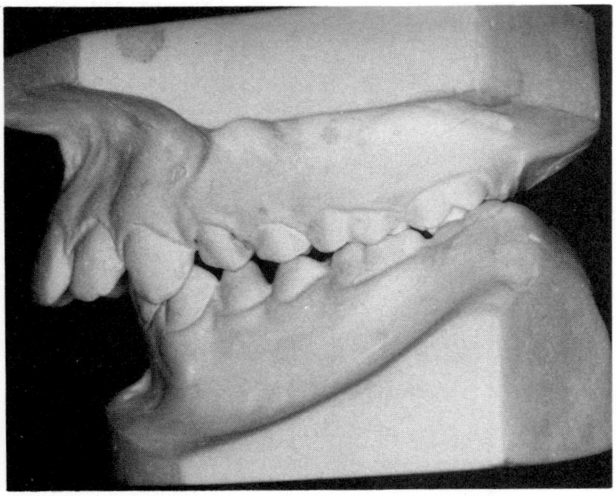

SR 12 years 8 months

NAME	SEX
S.R.	MALE

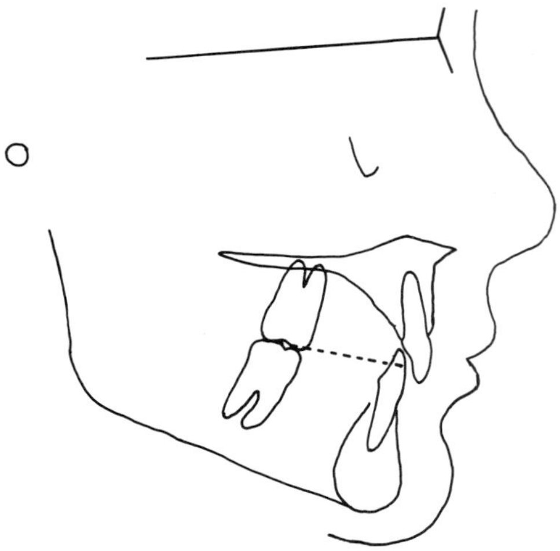

SKELETAL		
SNA	°	85.5
SNB	°	80.0
ANB	°	5.0
SN/MxP	°	3.0
MxP/MnP	°	23.5
LAFH	mm	59.5
UAFH	mm	47.5
LAFH/TAFH	%	55.5
LPFH	mm	43.5
UPFH	mm	47.0
PFH	mm	78.0
Wits	mm	1.5
TEETH		
Overjet	mm	4.5
Overbite	mm	7.0
UI/MxP	°	91.5
LI/MnP	°	87.5
IIangle	°	157.5
LI-APo	mm	−4.5
LI-NPo	mm	−2.5

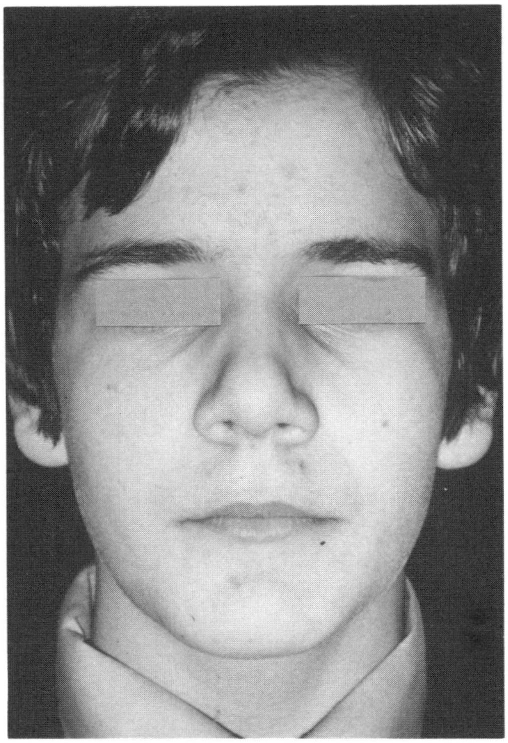

HISTORY

Reason for attendance

The parents were concerned about the proclined upper lateral incisors.

Dental history

The patient had received regular dental treatment. The lower right second deciduous molar had been lost at 9 years of age.

Medical history

There was no relevant medical history.

SOFT TISSUES

The lips were competent and the lip line was about halfway up the labial surfaces of the upper central incisors.

GENERAL CONDITION OF THE MOUTH

The oral hygiene was good.

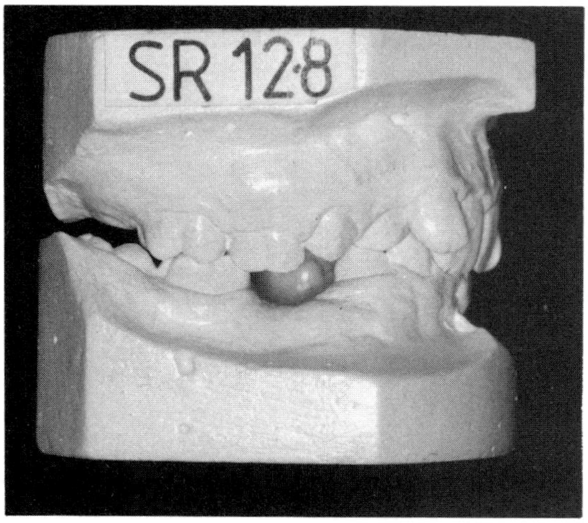

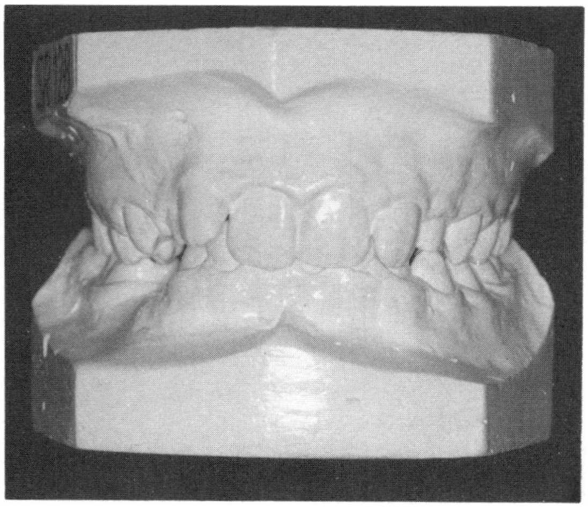

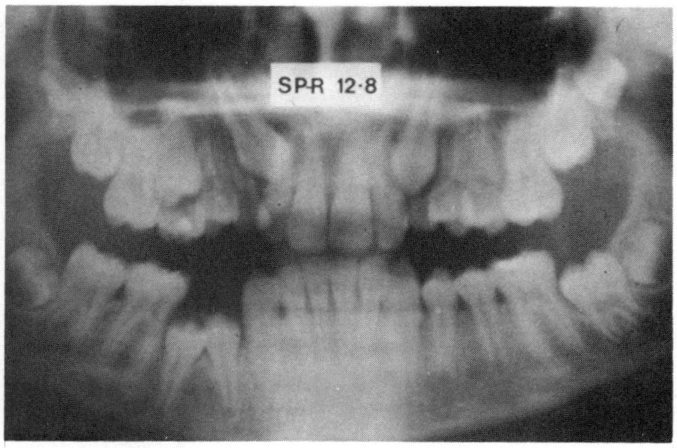
SP-R 12·8

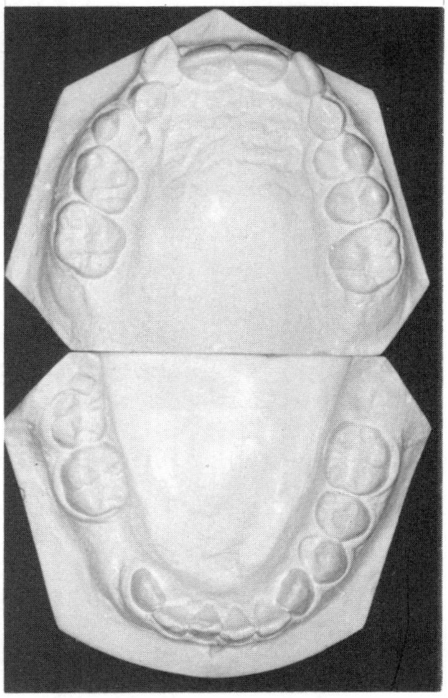

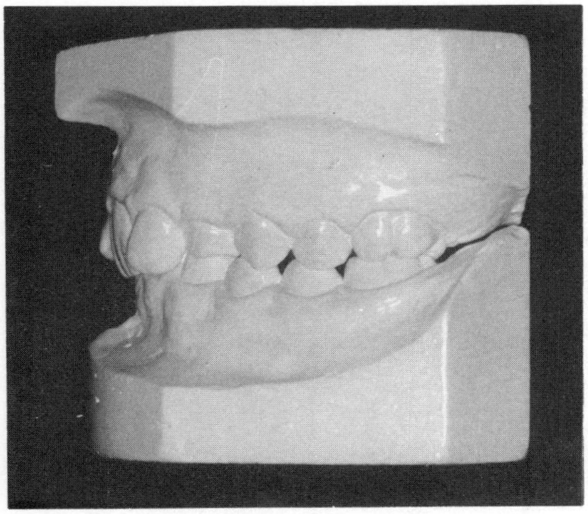

LM   12 years 1 month

NAME	SEX
L.M.	FEMALE

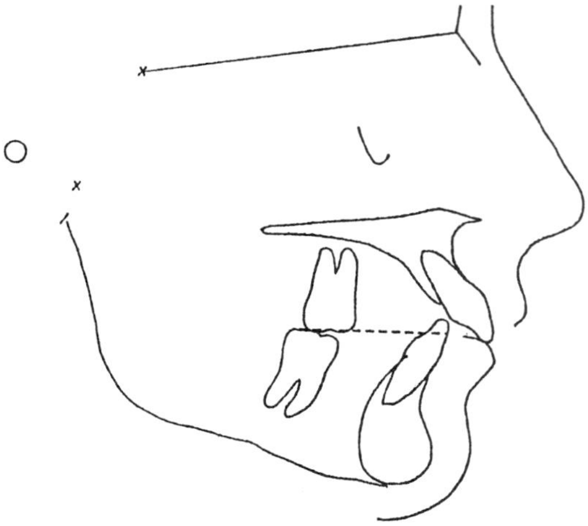

SKELETAL

SNA	°	81.5
SNB	°	77.5
ANB	°	4.0
SN/MxP	°	4.5
MxP/MnP	°	20.5
LAFH	mm	61.5
UAFH	mm	44.5
LAFH/TAFH	%	58.0
LPFH	mm	50.5
UPFH	mm	46.5
PFH	mm	78.0
Wits	mm	6.0

TEETH

Overjet	mm	9.5
Overbite	mm	6.5
UI/MxP	°	126.0
LI/MnP	°	109.5
IIangle	°	104.5
LI-APo	mm	0.5
LI-NPo	mm	1.5

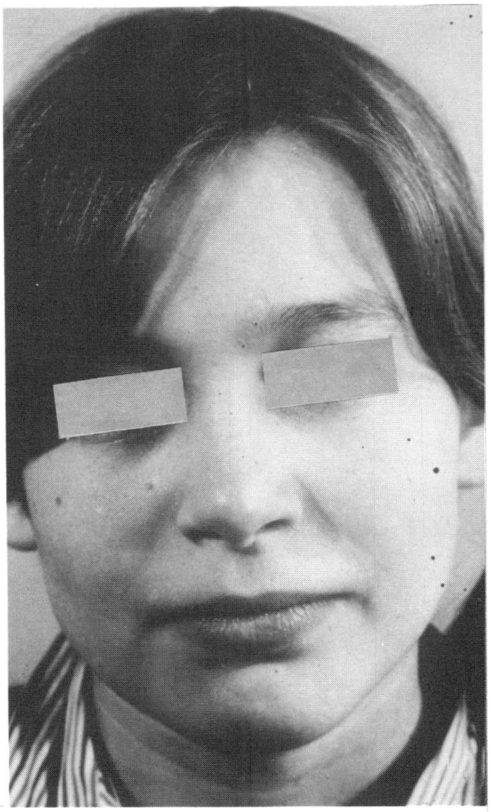

HISTORY

Reason for attendance

The patient reattended for review, having originally been seen a year earlier at the request of her general dental practitioner.

Dental history

When first seen at 11 years 1 month, a number of deciduous teeth were retained and the upper right deciduous molars and the lower right second deciduous molar were showing signs of submergence. Six months later the upper molars had been shed but the lower had become more seriously submerged and was therefore removed under local anaesthesia.

Medical history

There was no relevant medical history.

SOFT TISSUES

The lips were incompetent but habitually held together. The lower lip was just behind the upper incisor tips.

GENERAL CONDITION OF THE MOUTH

The oral hygiene was good.

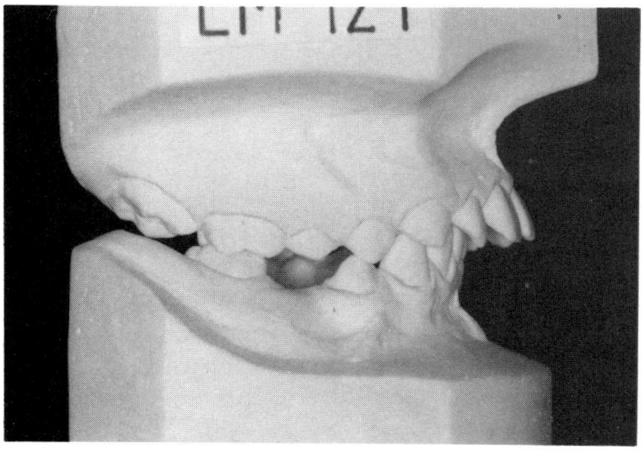

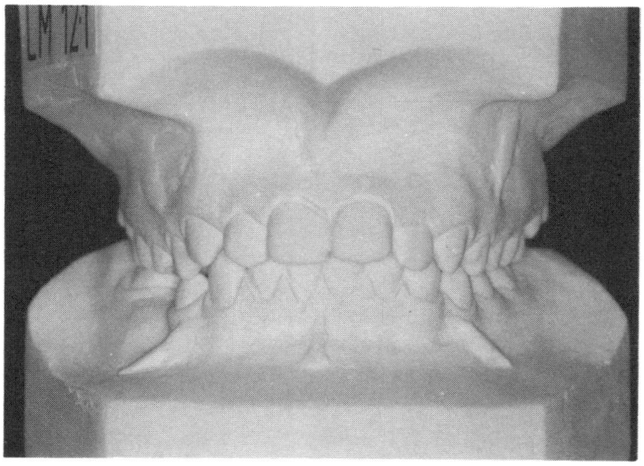

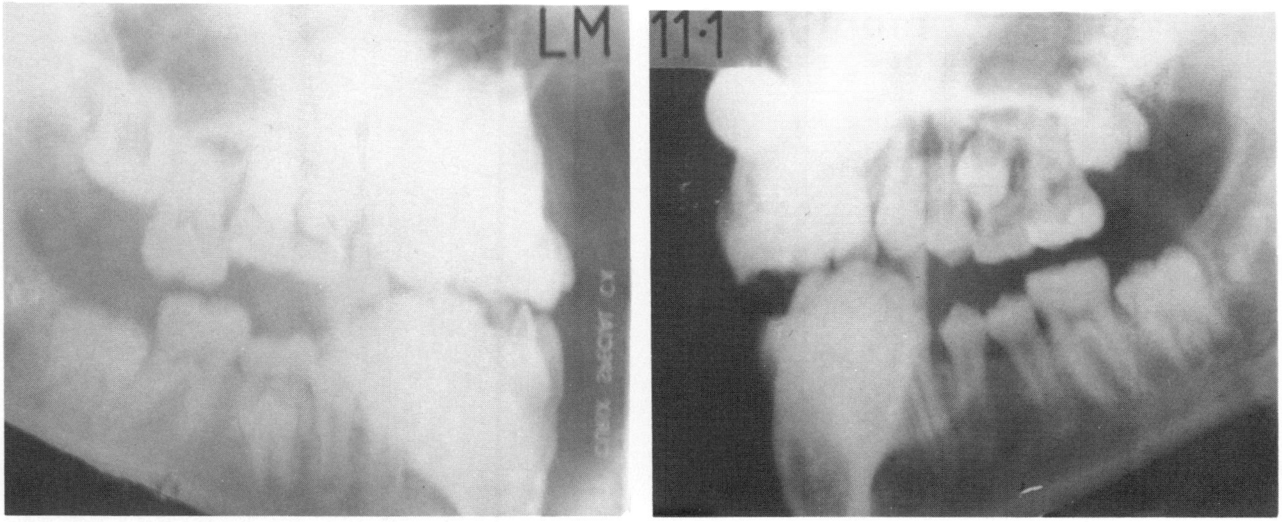
LM 11·1

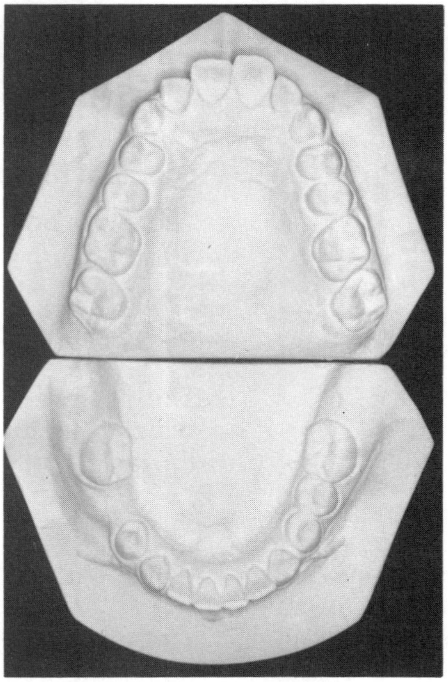

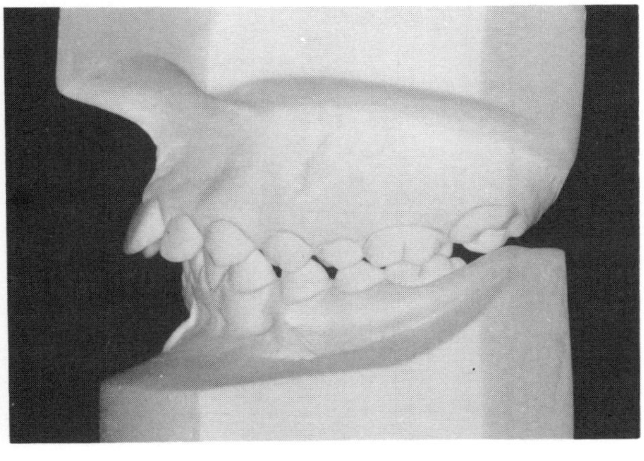

ML 10 years 1 month

NAME M.L.

SEX FEMALE

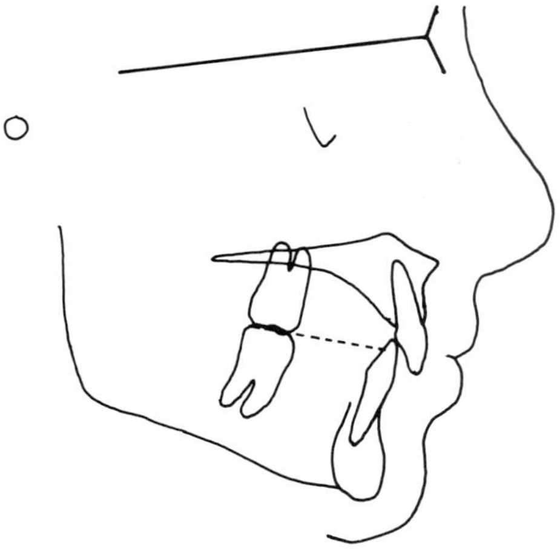

SKELETAL

SNA	°	83.5
SNB	°	76.5
ANB	°	7.0
SN/MxP	°	7.5
MxP/MnP	°	19.0
LAFH	mm	52.5
UAFH	mm	49.0
LAFH/TAFH	%	51.5
LPFH	mm	40.5
UPFH	mm	45.0
PFH	mm	71.5
Wits	mm	5.0

TEETH

Overjet	mm	6.5
Overbite	mm	7.5
UI/MxP	°	98.5
LI/MnP	°	93.0
IIangle	°	149.5
LI-APo	mm	-5.0
LI-NPo	mm	-1.5

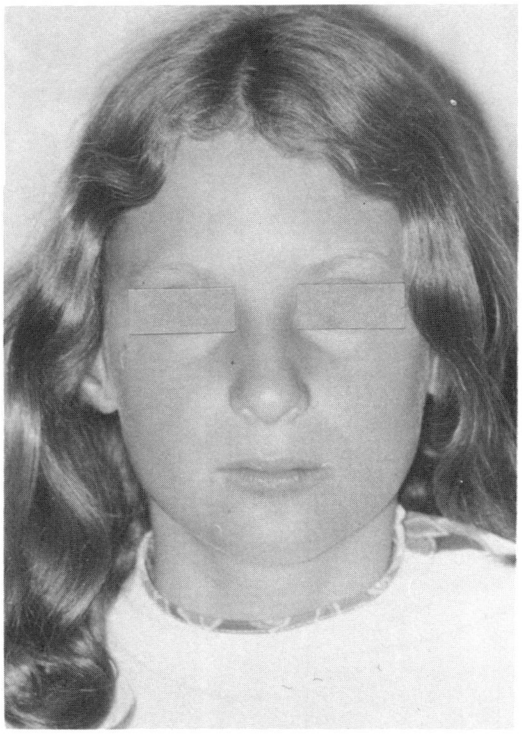

HISTORY

Reason for attendance

The patient attended the Primary Treatment Unit of the Dental School because her mother was concerned about the irregularity of her upper anterior teeth.

Dental history

Although nominally under the care of the Community Dental Service, ML appeared to have attended for little dental treatment apart from deciduous extractions. The patient was advised to seek routine dental care and subsequently decided to register with a local general dental practice.

Medical history

There was no relevant medical history.

SOFT TISSUES

The lips were competent and the lower lip, which was rather everted, rested halfway up the labial surfaces of the upper central incisors.

GENERAL CONDITION OF THE MOUTH

The oral hygiene was good and by the time treatment began she had a well cared for mouth.

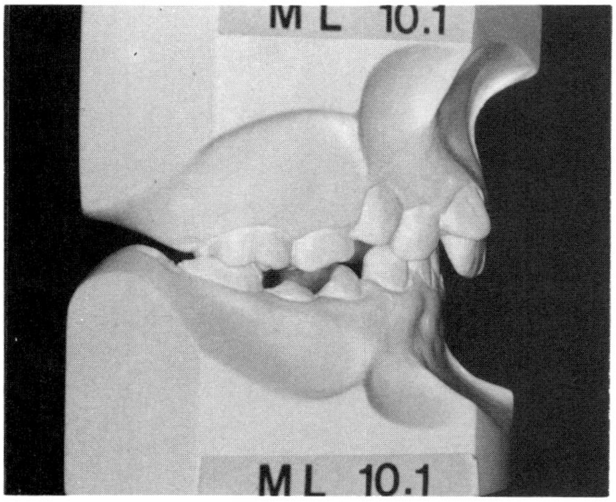

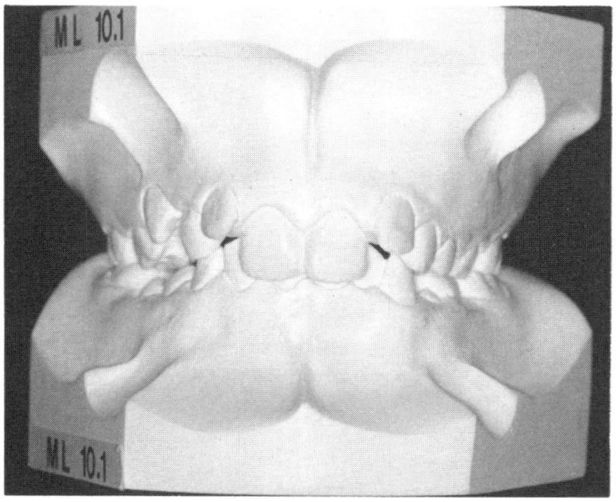

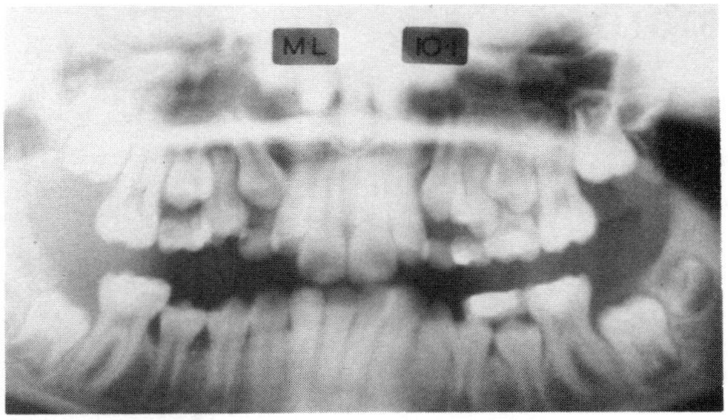
M.L.
10.1

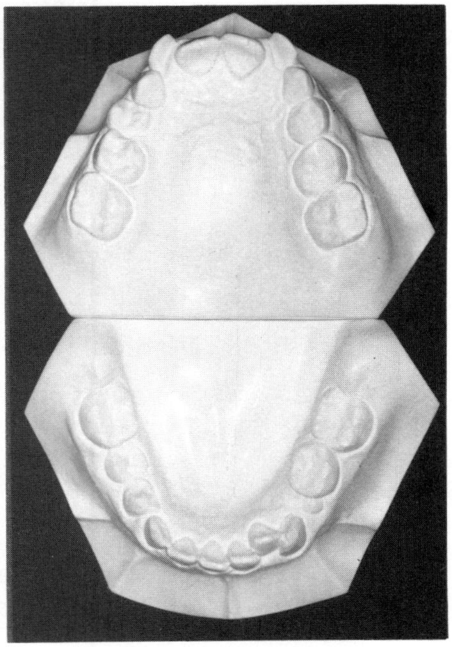

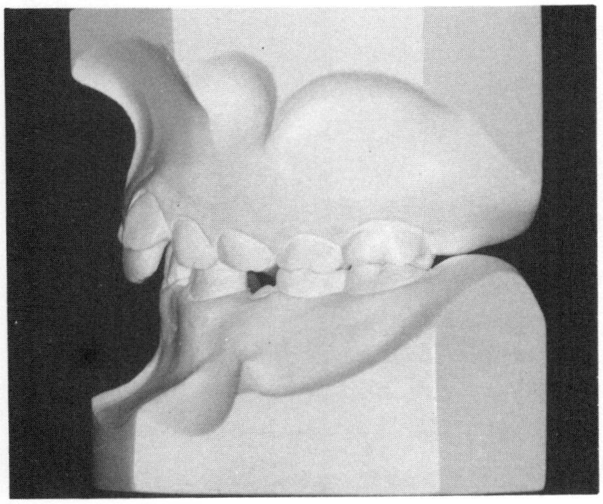

NO 14 years 4 months

NAME N.O.

SEX MALE

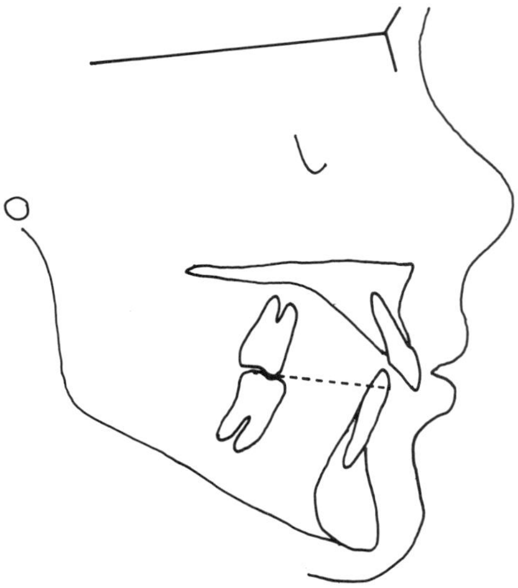

SKELETAL		
SNA	°	87.0
SNB	°	81.5
ANB	°	5.5
SN/MxP	°	4.5
MxP/MnP	°	28.0
LAFH	mm	67.0
UAFH	mm	54.5
LAFH/TAFH	%	55.0
LPFH	mm	40.5
UPFH	mm	53.5
PFH	mm	80.5
Wits	mm	4.0
TEETH		
Overjet	mm	7.5
Overbite	mm	4.0
UI/MxP	°	110.5
LI/MnP	°	86.5
IIangle	°	135.0
LI-APo	mm	-2.0
LI-NPo	mm	0.5

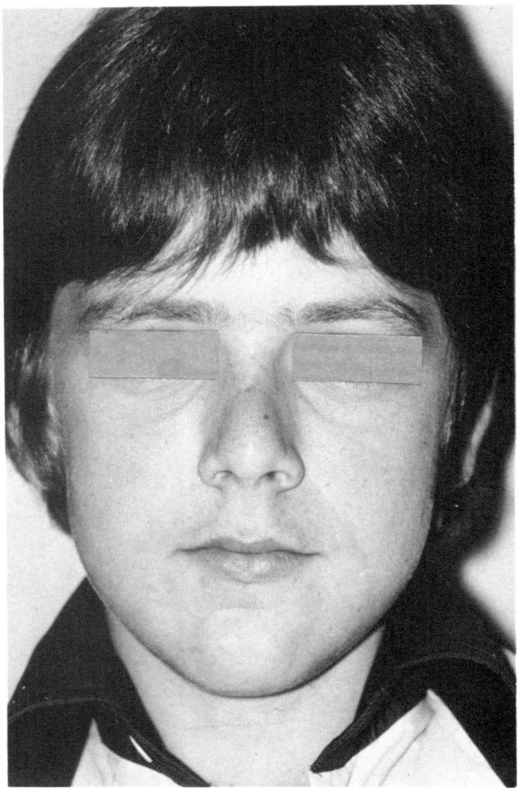

HISTORY

Reason for attendance

The patient had originally been seen at the request of the Community Dental Service. At that time the patient complained that his front teeth 'did not bite together very well'.

Dental history

There was no history of trauma to the upper anterior teeth, neither was there a digit-sucking habit.

Medical history

There was no relevant medical history.

SOFT TISSUES

The lips were competent and the lower lip rested about halfway up the labial surfaces of the upper central incisors.

GENERAL CONDITION OF THE MOUTH

The oral hygiene was good.

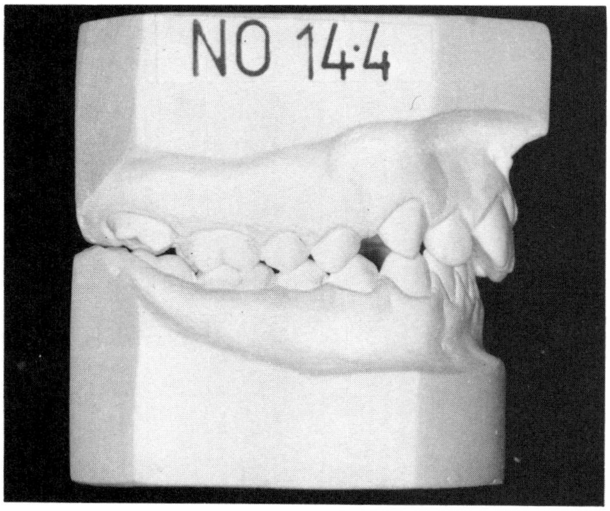

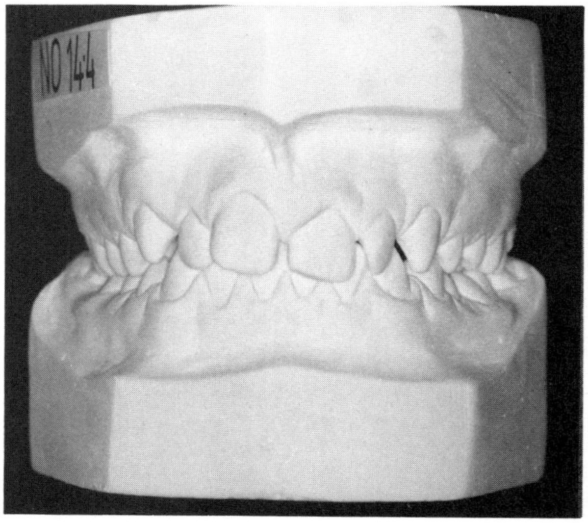

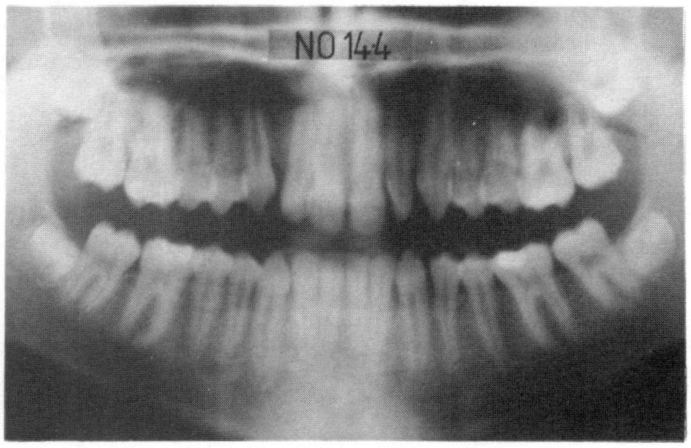
NO 144

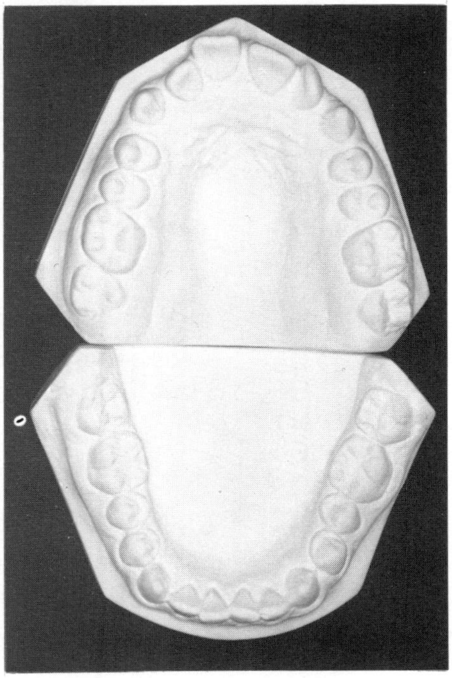

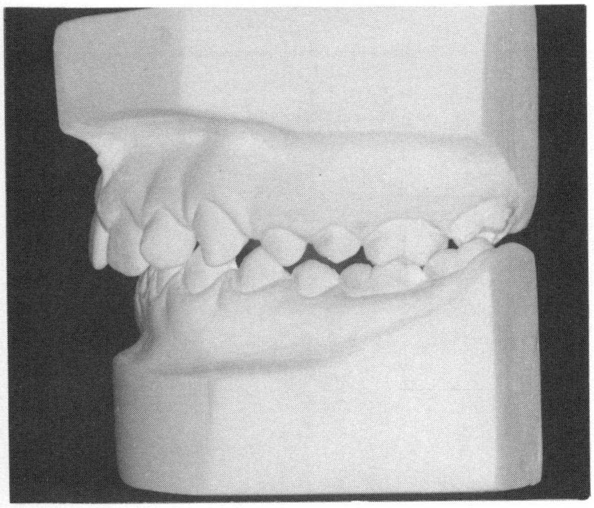

IR 13 years 7 months

NAME	SEX
I R	FEMALE

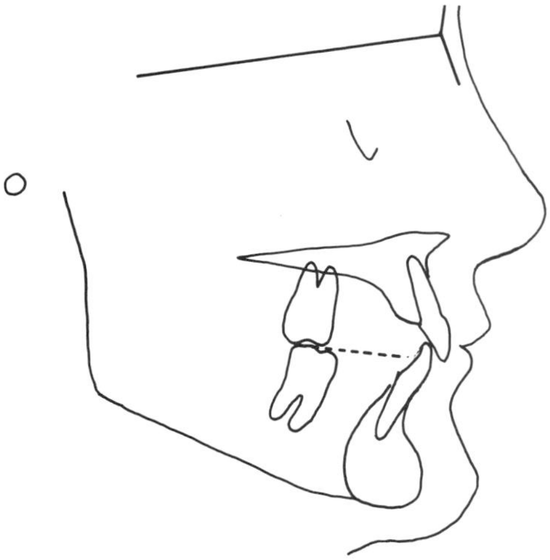

SKELETAL

SNA	°	79.0
SNB	°	77.0
ANB	°	2.0
SN/MxP	°	2.0
MxP/MnP	°	27.5
LAFH	mm	59.5
UAFH	mm	45.5
LAFH/TAFH	%	57.0
LPFH	mm	44.5
UPFH	mm	46.5
PFH	mm	72.5
Wits	mm	1.5

TEETH

Overjet	mm	4.5
Overbite	mm	2.5
UI/MxP	°	101.5
LI/MnP	°	95.0
IIangle	°	136.5
LI-APo	mm	-1.0
LI-NPo	mm	-2.0

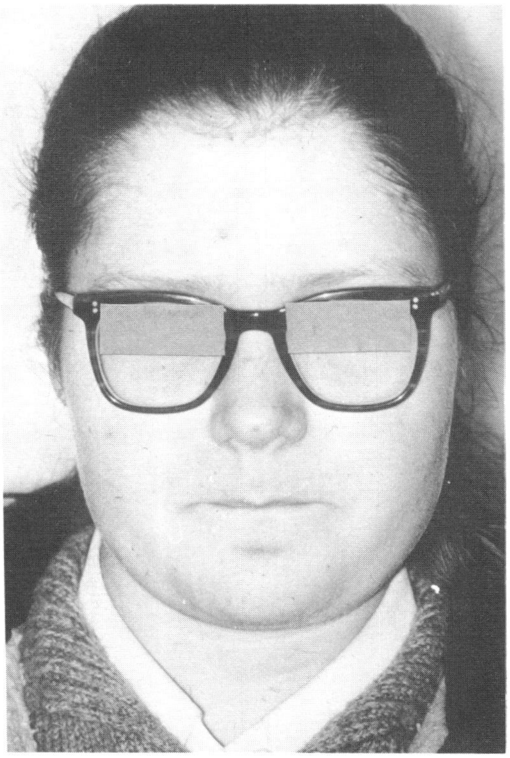

HISTORY

Reason for attendance

The patient was referred by her dental officer in the Community Dental Service for advice about her upper incisor irregularity.

Dental history

The patient had been a regular attender at the local community clinic since she was 8 years old.

Medical history

There was no relevant medical history.

Social history

The family lived 5 miles away and had no car but there was a good local bus service.

SOFT TISSUES

The lips were competent.

GENERAL CONDITION OF THE MOUTH

The oral hygiene was good.

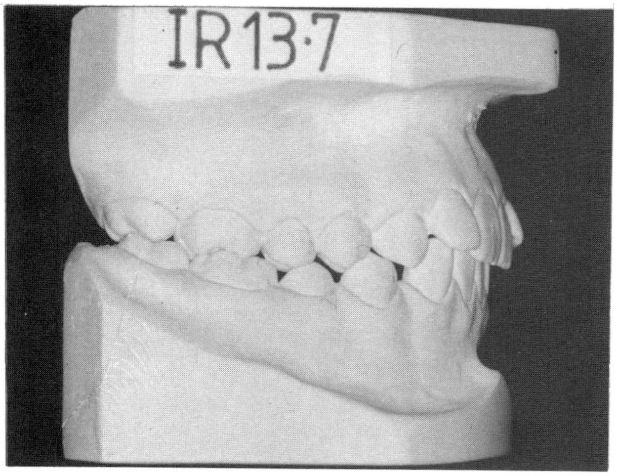

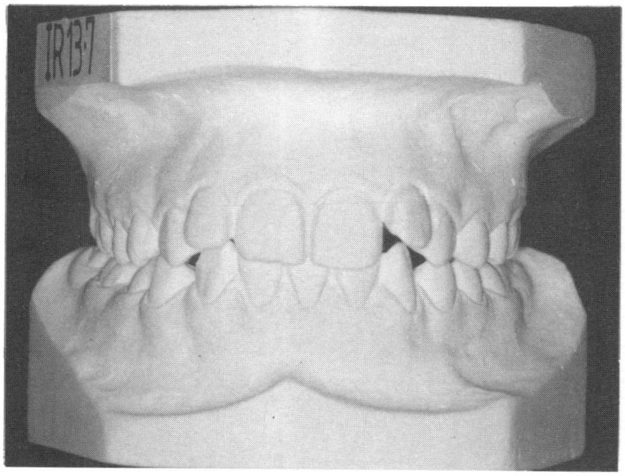

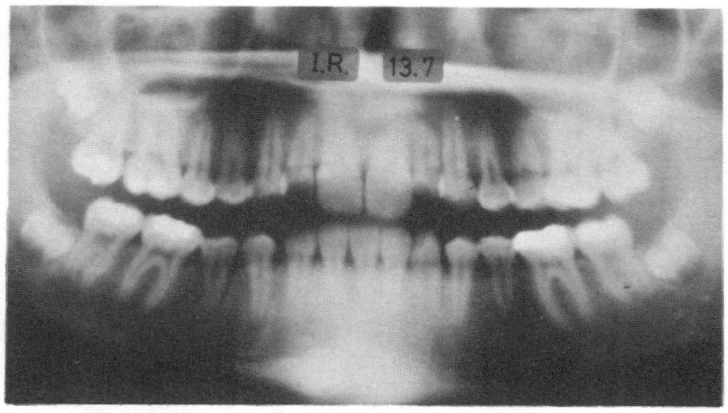
I.R.
13.7

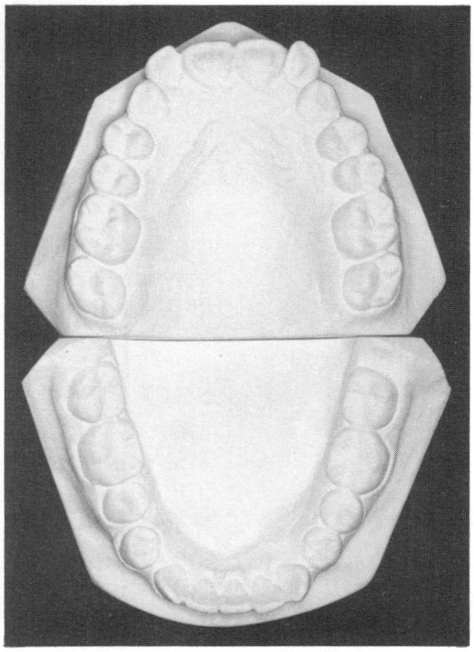

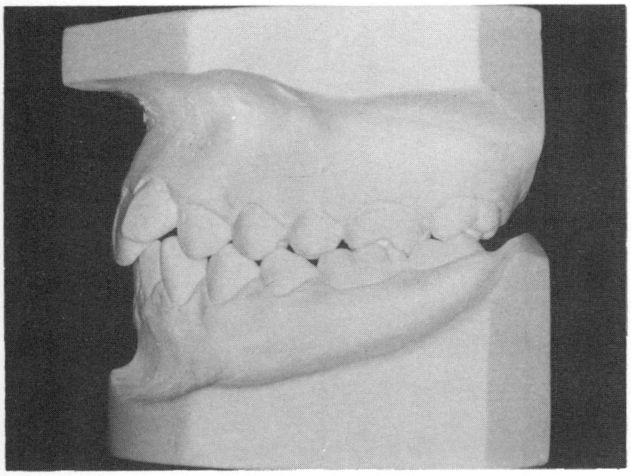

ATh 11 years 10 months

NAME A.Th.

SEX MALE

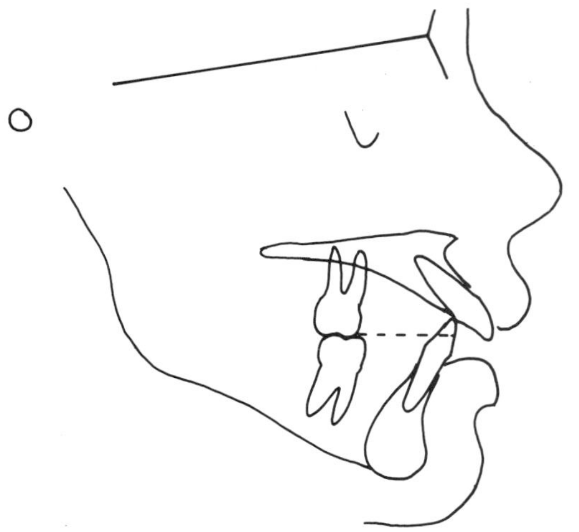

SKELETAL

SNA	°	84.5
SNB	°	80.0
ANB	°	5.0
SN/MxP	°	5.5
MxP/MnP	°	28.0
LAFH	mm	55.5
UAFH	mm	49.0
LAFH/TAFH	%	53.0
LPFH	mm	37.0
UPFH	mm	52.5
PFH	mm	67.0
Wits	mm	4.5

TEETH

Overjet	mm	8.5
Overbite	mm	3.5
UI/MxP	°	129.0
LI/MnP	°	97.5
IIangle	°	105.5
LI-APo	mm	4.0
LI-NPo	mm	6.0

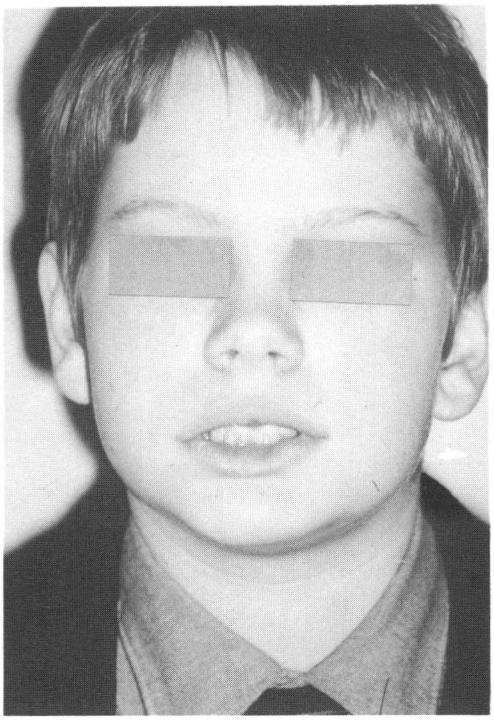

HISTORY

Reason for attendance

The patient was referred by his general dental practitioner for orthodontic treatment.

Dental history

The patient had attended the family practice since the age of 3 years.

Medical history

There was no relevant medical history.

Social history

The patient was attending a private preparatory school and lived with his grandmother during the term time as his parents lived and worked abroad. He joined his parents during the holidays, which were usually taken abroad.

SOFT TISSUES

The lips were potentially competent with the upper incisors trapped outside the lower lip. Note that the facial photograph is not typical of the resting posture. The patient still sucked his right thumb.

GENERAL CONDITION OF THE MOUTH

The oral hygiene was very poor and whilst the number of restorations was about average there was labial decalcification affecting all the upper incisors.

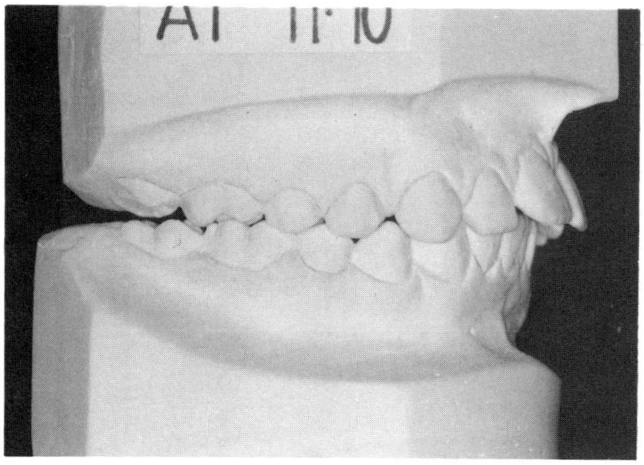

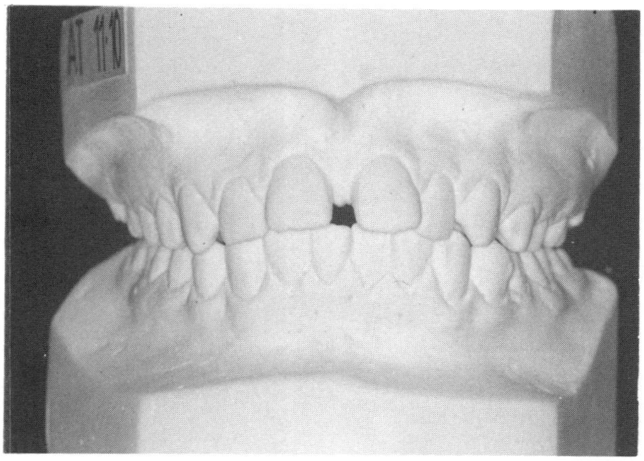

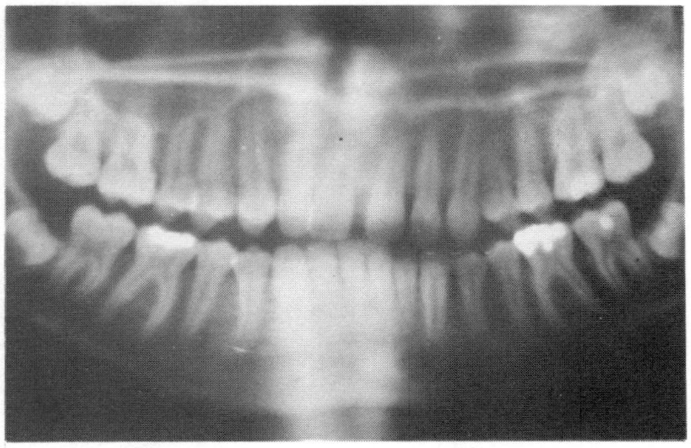

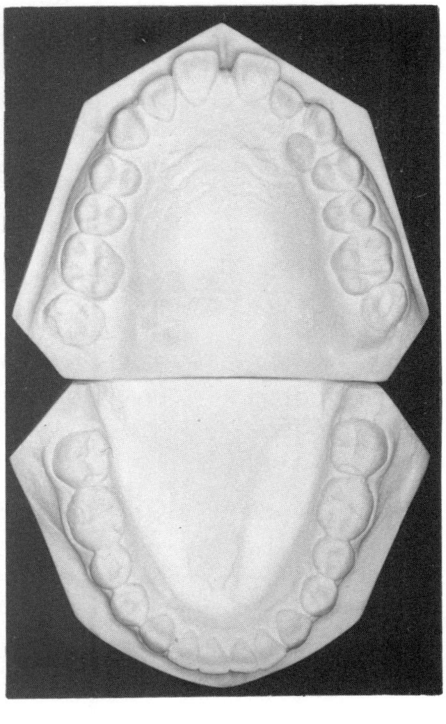

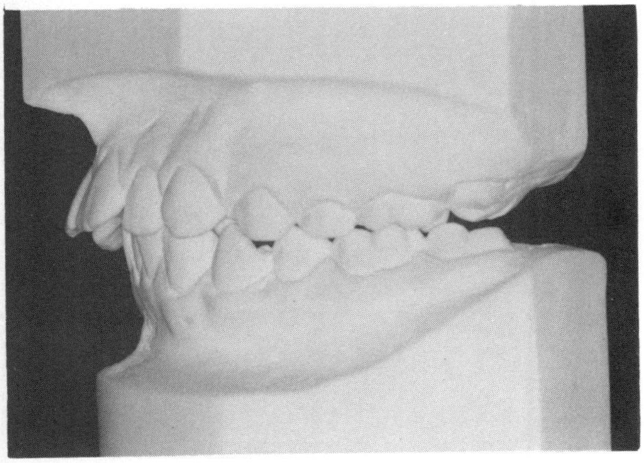

LJ 12 years 5 months

NAME L J   SEX FEMALE

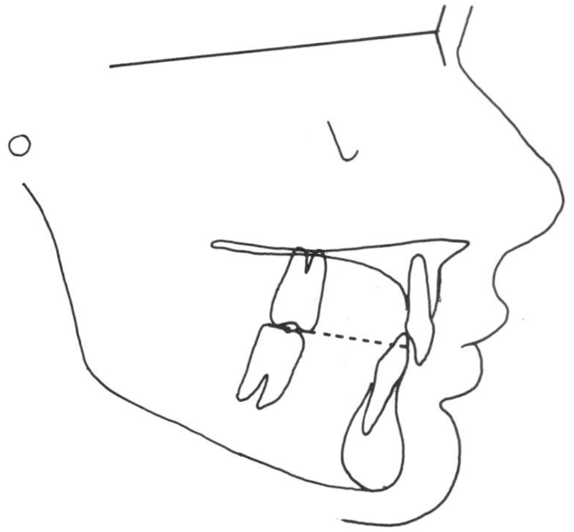

SKELETAL		
SNA	°	86.0
SNB	°	78.0
ANB	°	8.0
SN/MxP	°	5.0
MxP/MnP	°	21.0
LAFH	mm	56.5
UAFH	mm	48.5
LAFH/TAFH	%	54.0
LPFH	mm	40.0
UPFH	mm	47.0
PFH	mm	74.0
Wits	mm	5.5
TEETH		
Overjet	mm	3.5
Overbite	mm	6.5
UI/MxP	°	87.5
LI/MnP	°	97.0
IIangle	°	155.0
LI-APo	mm	-4.5
LI-NPo	mm	-1.0

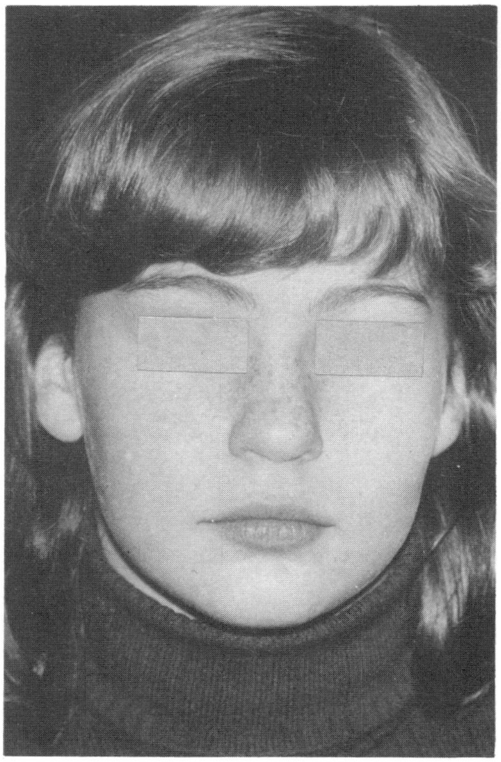

HISTORY

Reason for attendance

The patient had been referred by her general dental practitioner who had become concerned about the long-term effects of the very deep incisor overbite.

Dental history

The patient had always attended the family dental practice.

Medical history

There was no relevant medical history.

Social history

The patient attended a local public school as a weekly border. She was a keen musician and played the flute.

SOFT TISSUES

The lips were competent with the lower rather everted in form.

GENERAL CONDITION OF THE MOUTH

The oral hygiene was good.

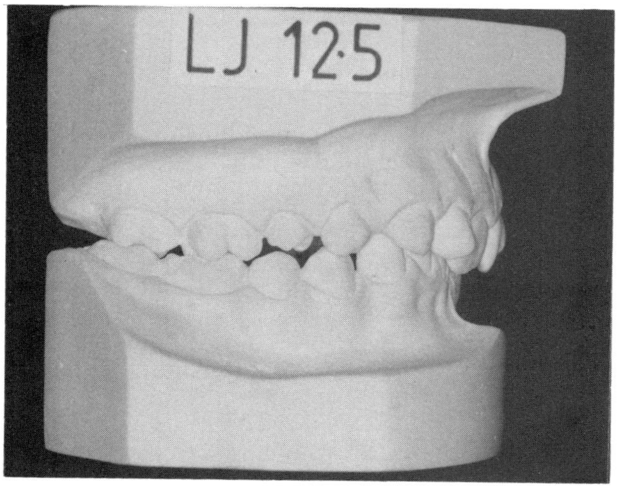

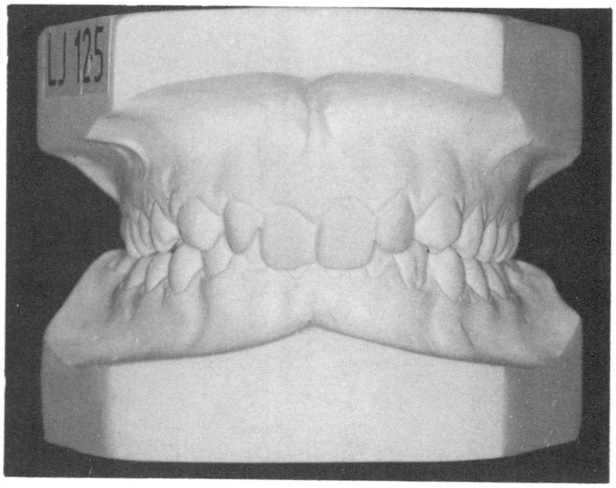

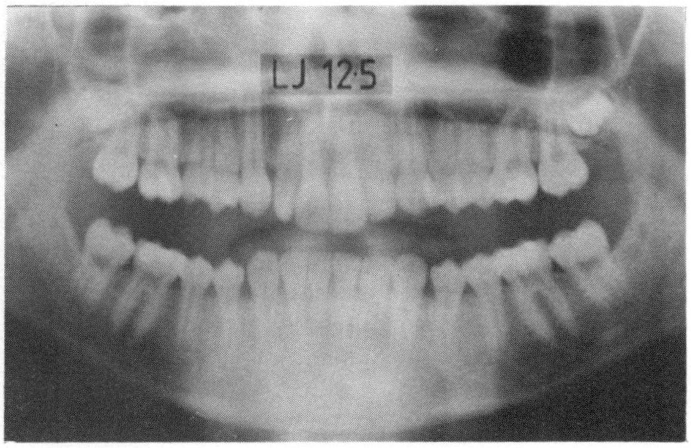
LJ 12·5

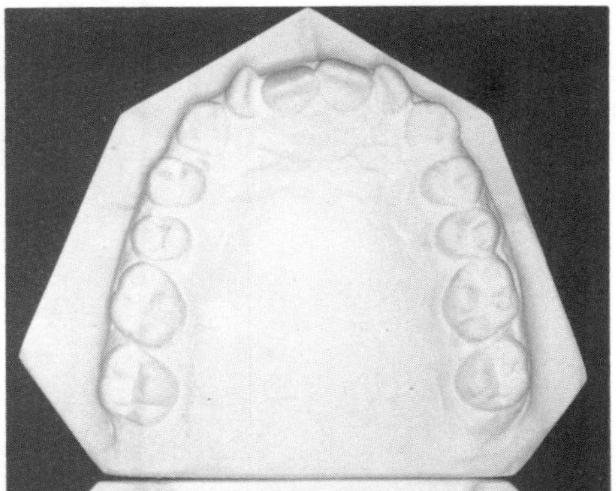

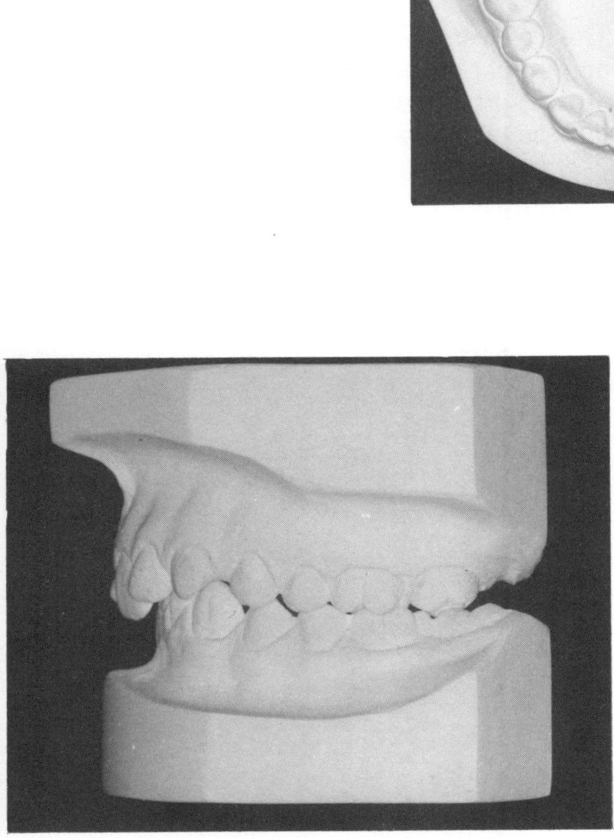

JS 12 years 6 months

NAME J S. SEX FEMALE

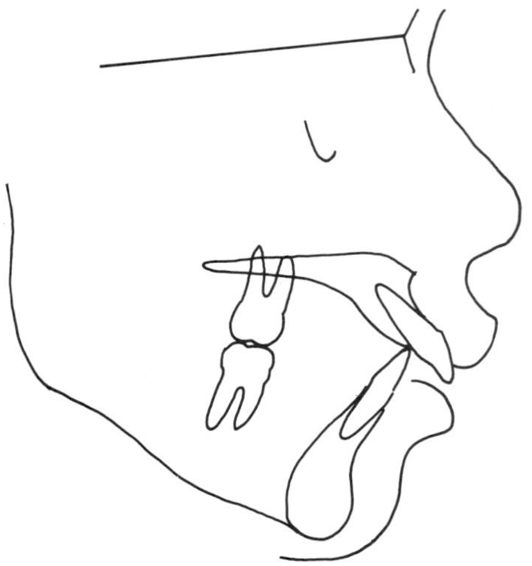

SKELETAL

SNA	°	85.0
SNB	°	77.0
ANB	°	8.0
SN/MxP	°	9.0
MxP/MnP	°	26.0
LAFH	mm	61.0
UAFH	mm	53.0
LAFH/TAFH	%	53.5
LPFH	mm	47.5
UPFH	mm	50.5
PFH	mm	72.0
Wits	mm	8.5

TEETH

Overjet	mm	11.5
Overbite	mm	5.5
UI/MxP	°	129.5
LI/MnP	°	97.5
IIangle	°	107.0
LI-APo	mm	2.5
LI-NPo	mm	7.5

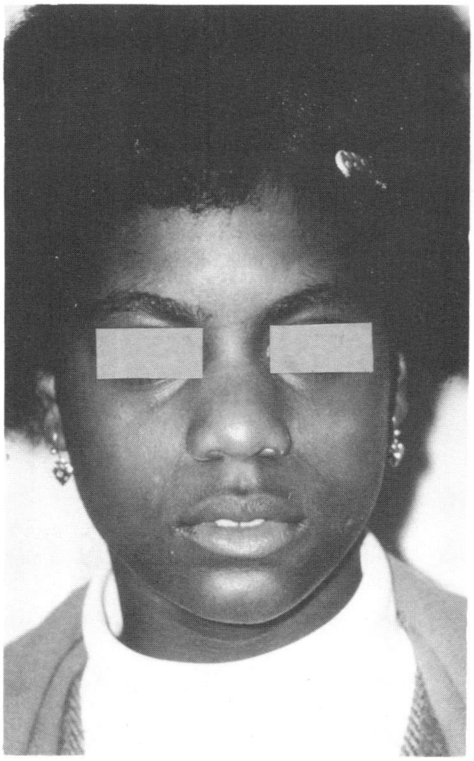

HISTORY

Reason for attendance

The patient was referred by a local Community Dental Officer for advice about the severely increased overjet.

Dental history

The patient had been seen by the Community Dental Service since the age of 8 years, although she was not a particularly regular attender.

Medical history

There was no relevant medical history.

SOFT TISSUES

The lips were incompetent and were habitually apart most of the time. The lower lip looked as if it would just control the upper incisor at rest if these teeth were retracted.

GENERAL CONDITION OF THE MOUTH

The oral hygiene was fair.

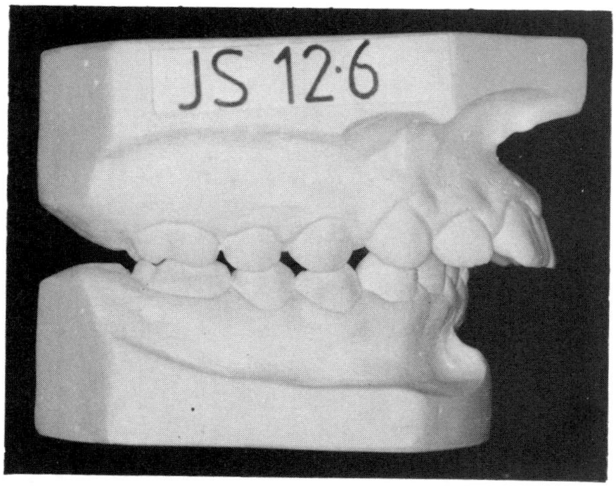

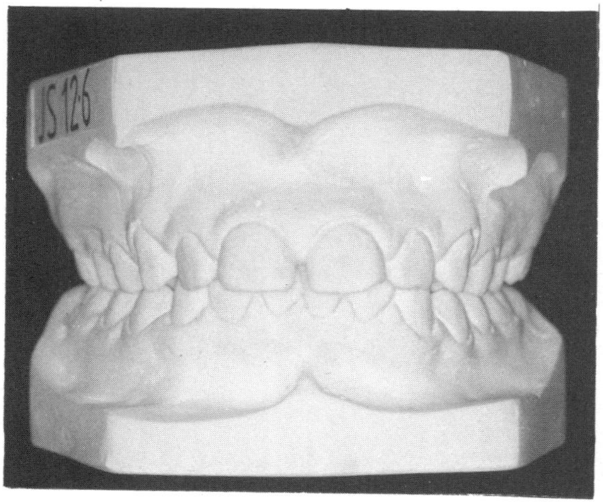

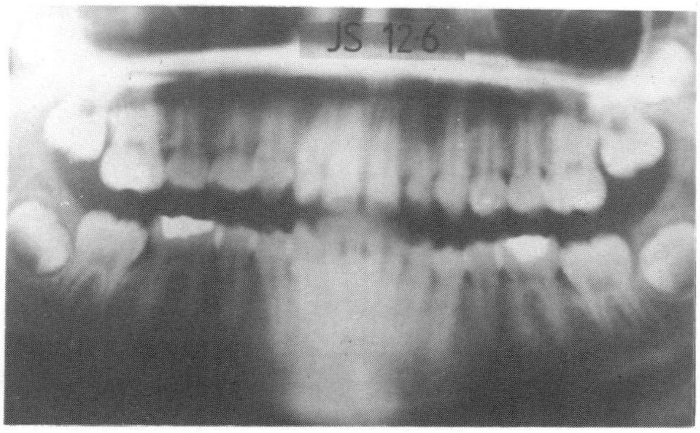
JS 12·6

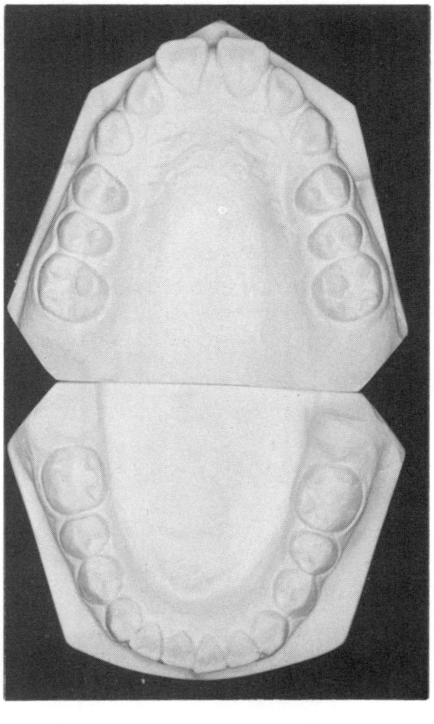

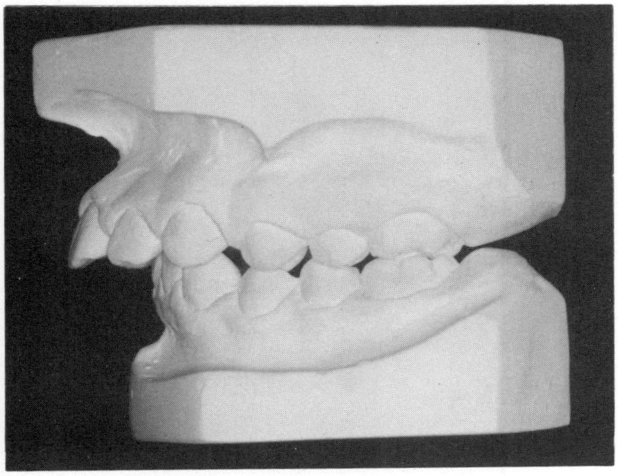

SECTION THREE

Case assessments

ONLY USE THIS SECTION WHEN YOU HAVE CARRIED OUT YOUR OWN ASSESSMENT. WITHOUT THIS INITIAL EFFORT YOU WILL LOSE MUCH OF THE TEACHING VALUE OF THIS TEXT.

After you have checked the details of your examination, plan the treatment using the guidelines given on the back cover. Your plan should be expressed in terms of treatment aims, treatment means and appliance design.

Note: As the cases assessments given here are those made at the time of the original clinical examination estimates of incisor angulation and skeletal pattern are sometimes at variance with the cephalometric findings.

Cases key

JB 10 years 3 months

HISTORY

Reason for attendance

The patient was referred by her father, a university lecturer who was dentally qualified. Both parents were concerned about the late appearance and palatal displacement of the upper right canine. The patient herself was slightly concerned about crowding in the upper labial region.

Dental history

The patient had taken fluoride tablets from birth and had never had any dental treatment apart from removal of a mucous retention cyst carried out under local anaesthesia at 7 years.

Medical history

There was no relevant medical history.

EXAMINATION

Extraoral

The patient had near normal sagittal jaw relationship and an average lower face height. The lips were mildly incompetent but habitually held together. The lower lip at rest just covered the upper incisal edges.

Intraoral

General condition of the mouth
The patient had an excellent caries free mouth with good oral hygiene and was dentally rather advanced for her age.

The *lower incisors* were of average inclination and very slightly crowded.

The *lower canines* were slighty distally inclined and the lower left canine was slightly short of space.

The *lower buccal segments* were well aligned.

The *upper incisors* were of average inclination. The upper right lateral was mildly crowded and displaced labially. Both upper lateral incisors were rather small.

The *upper left canine* was mesially inclined and slightly short of space. The upper right was mesially inclined and crowded palatally.

The *upper buccal segments* were well aligned with the upper second molars just appearing in the mouth.

With the teeth in occlusion there was a Class I incisor relationship with average overjet and overbite except on the upper right lateral incisor where there was a local open bite. The upper right canine was in palatal crossbite. The buccal segments were almost Class I on the left and a half-unit Class II on the right.

Radiographic

All teeth were present, including the third molars in all quadrants. There was evidence of upper molar 'stacking'.

Cephalometric

The cephalometric tracing confirmed that the patient had a skeletal 1 dental base relationship (ANB 3°). The maxillary/mandibular planes angle was slightly below average (24°) and the lower face height was 58 mm. The upper and lower incisors were of average inclination to their respective planes.

LB 23 years 3 months

HISTORY

Reason for attendance

The patient was a third-year dental student who was quite happy with her appearance but had become concerned with the overeruption of the lower right second molar and the widening of the periodontal space of the lower right first molar which she judged to be due to the traumatic occlusion with the upper left second molar.

Dental history

She had received routine dental treatment for many years and had just completed having all past restorations replaced by a member of staff.

Medical history

There was no relevant medical history.

EXAMINATION

Extraoral

There was a mild skeletal 2 dental base relationship and a slightly reduced lower face height and Frankfort/mandibular planes angle.

The lips were mildly incompetent but habitually held together. At rest the lower lip just covered the upper incisor tips.

Intraoral

General condition of the mouth
The oral hygiene was good but the teeth were heavily restored.

The *lower incisors* were slightly proclined and well aligned. The lower left central incisor had a porcelain jacket crown.

The *lower canines* were upright and well aligned.

The *lower buccal segments*: both lower first molars were heavily restored and the occlusal surface of the unopposed lower right second molar was 1.5–2 mm above the level of the occlusal plane.

The *upper incisors*: the central incisors appeared to be slightly retroclined but the upper laterals were crowded slightly labially and mesiolabially rotated.

The *upper canines* were upright and well aligned.

The *upper buccal segments* were uncrowded. The upper right first molar had been lost and the upper second molar in this quadrant had moved forwards and had rotated mesiopalatally into contact with the second premolar.

With the teeth in occlusion the incisor relationship was on the border between Class I and Class II division 2. The overjet was 2.5 mm and the overbite slightly increased and complete. The canine occlusion was Class I on the right and very slightly Class II on the left. The molar occlusion was almost Class I on the right but a half-unit Class II on the left. The lower right second molar was unopposed and had overerupted.

Radiographic

All four third molars were absent. There was evidence of slight bone loss mesial to the upper right second molar and slight widening of the periodontal membrane on the distal surface of the mesial root of the lower right first molar.

Cephalometric

Examination showed that the skeletal 2 dental base relationship was more marked than the clinical examination had suggested. The SNA was 76°, hence the corrected ANB angle was 7°. The lower incisors were markedly proclined (103.5° to MdP) and the uppers severely retroclined (89° to MxP).

CB 10 years 1 month

HISTORY

Reason for attendance

The patient had been referred by her general dental practitioner because, despite her age, both CB and her mother were keen for treatment to begin to correct the prominence of the upper incisors. Her mother had had multibanded fixed appliance treatment as a child and CB was well aware of what orthodontic treatment would probably entail.

Dental history

CB had been a regular attender with the family dental practitioner for several years.

Medical history

There was no relevant medical history.

EXAMINATION

Extraoral

CB had a marked class 2 dental base relationship and a raised Frankfort/mandibular planes angle. The lips were grossly incompetent and habitually apart. At rest the lower lip lay just behind the upper incisor tips whilst the upper lip line was level with the gingival margins of the upper incisors. There was no history of a digit-sucking habit.

Intraoral

General condition of the mouth
The patient was in the mixed dentition stage. The oral hygiene was good and the caries rate low.

The *lower incisors* were of average inclination to the mandibular plane and severely crowded. The lower left central incisor was crowded labially and largely excluded from the arch and the lower left lateral was lingually displaced. Both lateral incisors were slightly distally inclined.

The *lower right canine* was upright and the *lower left* mesially inclined. Both canines were crowded and slightly buccally placed.

The *lower buccal segments* were uncrowded.

Upper incisors: the upper central incisors were slightly proclined and the upper lateral incisors, although of normal angulation, were crowded.

The *upper canines* were both mesially inclined and crowded. The upper left was slightly buccally placed, while the upper right was partly erupted.

The *upper buccal segments* were uncrowded.

With the teeth in occlusion there was a marked Class II division 1 incisor occlusion with an overjet of 13 mm. The overbite was increased and complete against the palate but there was no sign of soft tissue trauma. The centrelines coincided. The buccal segments were a half-unit Class II on the left and a full unit Class II on the right.

Radiographic

All successional teeth were present on x-ray and there was early evidence of development of all third molars. All first deciduous molars showed signs of root resorption and the lower left appeared to be near to exfoliation.

Cephalometric

The cephalometric findings confirmed that the patient had a marked skeletal Class 2 base relationship. There was an ANB angle of 6.5° (corrected 5.5°). The maxillary/mandibular planes angle was raised at 32° and the lower face height was increased to 67 mm . The upper incisors were proclined at 115° to the maxillary plane but after due allowance was made for the raised maxillary/mandibular planes angle, the lower incisors were found to be of average inclination.

AT 13 years 2 months

HISTORY

Reason for attendance

The patient was referred by her general dental practitioner for treatment of her lower incisor crowding, about which she was not greatly concerned.

Dental history

She had received regular dental treatment from the age of 6 years. She reported that the lower left second molar was giving her intermittent pain.

Medical history

There was no relevant medical history.

EXAMINATION

Extraoral

The patient appeared to have a very mild skeletal Class 2 dental base relationship. The Frankfort/mandibular planes angle was average, as was the lower face height. The lips were competent.

Intraoral

General condition of the mouth
The oral hygiene was only fair. The caries experience was about average although there was a large amalgam restoration in the partially erupted lower left second molar.

The *lower incisors* were proclined and slightly crowded. There was supplemental lower incisor, probably the tooth in the midline, and this accounted for both the crowding in this region and the 'fanning' of the adjacent incisors.

The *lower canines* were both upright and well aligned.

The *lower buccal segments*: the left was well aligned except for a slight rotation of the second premolar. The lower right was slightly crowded with the second premolar buccally displaced.

The *upper incisors* were of normal angulation and slightly crowded. The upper left central incisor was slightly distolabially rotated and the left lateral incisor had a marked mesiolabial rotation.

The *upper canines* were slightly mesially inclined and well aligned.

The *upper buccal segments* were generally well aligned but the upper right second premolar was rotated through 180°.

With the teeth in occlusion there was a Class I incisor relationship with an overjet of 4 mm and an average and complete overbite. Because of the supplemental incisor it was not possible to determine the centreline relationship. The buccal occlusion was a full unit Class II on both sides and the upper right second premolar was in crossbite.

Radiographic

The lower left second molar had recurrent caries beneath its large restoration and there appeared to be a periapical area on the mesial root. All third molars were present and well placed, although the upper right was rather small.

Cephalometric

At first sight the mild skeletal 2 dental base relationship was confirmed by an ANB angle of 5.5°. However the raised SNA of 87° gives a corrected ANB of 2.5°. The upper incisors were of average inclination (112° to the maxillary plane) and the lower incisors markedly proclined at 102° to the mandibular plane. The maxillary/mandibular planes angle (18°) was slightly below average, as was the lower face height (59.5 mm).

CW 11 years 11 months

HISTORY

Reason for attendance

The family had recently moved to the area. The patient and her mother were concerned about soreness to the gum behind the upper central incisors.

Dental history

The family were regular dental attenders. CW had her upper deciduous central incisors avulsed at age 18 months.

Medical history

There was no relevant medical history.

Social history

The family lived 12 miles away and have a car, although the patient is quite badly travel-sick.

EXAMINATION

Extraoral

The anteroposterior jaw relationship was skeletal Class 2 (moderately severe) with reduced lower face height and Frankfort/mandibular planes angle. There was no facial asymmetry. The lips were mildly competent, habitually held together with the upper incisors trapped between them.

Intraoral

General condition of the mouth
The oral hygiene was good and the caries rate average.

The *lower incisors* were of average inclination, slightly crowded with the midline slightly displaced to the right.

The *lower canines* were both distally inclined with the lower left markedly so, with an associated distolabial rotation. The left canine was slightly short of space.

The *buccal segments* were crowded with both the lower second premolars lingually displaced.

The *upper incisors* were proclined and slightly spaced with their centreline displaced to the left.

The *upper canines* were of normal angulation and well aligned.

The *upper buccal segments*: both first premolars were slightly buccally displaced.

With the teeth in occlusion the upper incisors had a Class II division 1 relationship. The overjet was 11 mm and there was a deep and complete overbite. There was evidence of palatal trauma (indentation and blanching) but no apparent bone loss. The canines were a full unit Class II on both sides. The molar occlusion was half a unit Class II on both sides and the upper first premolars were in buccal occlusion. There was no mandibular displacement.

Radiographic

All teeth including third molars were present and of good form although the roots of all the teeth, particularly the upper central incisors, appeared to be rather short.

Cephalometric

The patient had a skeletal Class 2 dental base relationship with an ANB angle of 5°. (The correction for the raised angle SNA does not give an appropriate result in this case. Consideration of this point is outside the scope of the present text.)

The upper incisors were moderately proclined (120° to Mx) and the lower incisors were at about average inclination if account is taken of the reduced maxillary/mandibular planes angle (24.5°). The lower face height (54 mm) is 1 s.d. below the mean for a child of this age and sex.

RP 9 years 9 months

HISTORY

Reason for attendance

The patient had originally attended at 7 years of age, referred by her general dental practitioner because the patient's mother was concerned about very severe lower anterior crowding. The extraction of all four deciduous canines was advised.

Dental history

The patient had received regular dental treatment from an early age.

Medical history

There was no relevant medical history.

EXAMINATION

Extraoral

The patient appeared to have a Class 1 or mild skeletal 2 dental base relationship with an average face height. The lips were competent and there was an average lip line (the lower lip rested one third of the way up the labial surface of the upper incisors).

Intraoral

General condition of the mouth
The oral hygiene was good and the caries experience average for the patient's age.

The *lower incisors* were retroclined to the mandibular plane and very slightly crowded.

The *lower canines*: the lower left was upright and the lower right mesially inclined. Both were slightly crowded and buccally displaced.

The *lower buccal segments* were well aligned.

The *upper incisors* were of near average inclination and spaced.

The *upper canines* were palpable buccally and appeared to be rather upright on x-ray. Both teeth were short of space – the left severely so.

The *upper buccal segments* were well aligned, with the possible exception of the partially erupted upper right first premolar which appeared to be slightly rotated.

With the teeth in occlusion there was a Class I incisor relationship with an average overjet and average and complete overbite. (The appearance of a reduced overbite on the models is due to the imminent shedding of the lower left deciduous first molar.) The upper left lateral was almost in crossbite with the buccally displaced lower canine. The upper and lower centrelines were coincident with each other and the midline of the face. The buccal occlusion was almost Class I on the left and right.

Radiographic

All teeth were developing normally with the exception of the third molar, signs of which would be unusual in any case at this age. There was little evidence of molar stacking and first molars had minimal restorations (lower) or very early cavities (upper).

Cephalometric

The cephalometric tracing does at first sight confirm the clinical appearance but after allowance has been made for the low SNA angle (74°) the patient can be seen to have a mild skeletal 2 dental base relationship (ANB 1° corrected = 4.5°). Both upper and lower incisors are slightly retroclined. Both the lower face height and maxillary/mandibular planes angle are within normal limits.

SD 11 years 4 months

HISTORY

Reason for attendance

The patient was referred by her general dental practitioner who had noticed that the upper right lateral incisor had erupted into crossbite. The patient and parent were unconcerned.

Dental history

Although under the care of her family practitioner the patient was caries-free and at the time of first attending had never received any dental treatment apart from examinations.

Medical history

There was no relevant medical history.

EXAMINATION

Extraoral

The patient had a skeletal 1 dental base relationship and an average face height. There was no evidence of facial asymmetry. The lips were competent.

Intraoral

General condition of the mouth
The dentition was in the early mixed dentition stage (i.e. the patient was very late in her dental development). The oral hygiene was excellent and the mouth was caries free.

The *lower incisors* were of normal angulation, well aligned with spacing distal to the lateral incisors.

The *lower canines* were unerupted.

The *lower buccal segments* were well aligned.

The *upper incisors*: there was a marked median diastema but despite this space both upper lateral incisors were mesiolabially rotated and rather small. The right lateral was in crossbite.

The *upper canines* were unerupted and not yet palpable.

The *upper buccal segments* were well aligned.

With the teeth in occlusion the incisor relationship was Class I. The overjet was 3 mm and the overbite average on the centrals but reduced on both laterals. The centreline in the lower arch was to the right and this was aggravated by a small displacement from an initial contact on the upper right lateral incisor. The molar occlusion was Class I on the left and a full unit Class II on the right.

Radiographic

All teeth apart from third molars were present on x-ray. The orthopantomogram confirmed that the patient was generally late in her dental development by about 2 years.

Cephalometric

The tracing confirmed the clinical impression. There was skeletal 1 sagittal jaw relationship (ANB 4° corrected = 2°) and an average maxillary/mandibular planes angle and lower anterior face height. Both the upper and lower incisors were very slightly retroclined to their respective planes (103.5; 89.5°).

JK 11 years 7 months

HISTORY

Reason for attendance

The patient had been referred by his general practitioner, a dental officer in the Community Dental Service. The boy was not unduly concerned about his malocclusion but accepted the idea of simple treatment.

Dental history

The patient had received routine dental treatment from the age of 5 years.

Medical history

There was no relevant medical history.

EXAMINATION

Extraoral

JK had a near ideal dental base relationship and an average lower face height. The lips were slightly incompetent but held together some of the time.

Intraoral

General condition of the mouth
The oral hygiene was good and the caries rate average.

The *lower incisors* were proclined – the central incisors particularly so – and moderately crowded.

The *lower canines* were mesially inclined. The lower left canine was slightly distolabially rotated and slightly crowded.

The *lower buccal segments*: the lower second premolars were both slightly short of space and partially erupted.

The *upper incisors* were of average inclination and slightly crowded. Both central incisors were slightly distolabially rotated.

The *upper canines* were mesially inclined, slightly crowded and mesiolabially rotated.

The *upper buccal segments* were generally well aligned although both first premolars were very slightly rotated.

With the teeth in occlusion there was a very mild Class II division 1 incisor relationship. The overjet was 5 mm and the overbite slightly increased and complete. The molar occlusion was Class I on both sides.

Radiographic

All teeth were present, including third molars and there was no evidence of any pathology.

Cephalometric

Analysis confirmed the skeletal 1 dental base relationship with an ANB of 4.0° (corrected 3°). The maxillary/mandibular planes angle was slightly raised. The upper incisors were of near ideal angulation (112° to MxP) and the lowers were slightly proclined (102° to MdP).

JA 10 years 5 months

HISTORY

Reason for attendance

The patient's general practitioner was concerned about the developing Class III incisor relationship.

Dental history

The patient had received routine treatment from the family practitioner. This included extraction under local anaesthesia. There was a history of poor dietary control of fermentable carbohydrate but this had been corrected.

Medical history

There was no relevant medical history.

EXAMINATION

Extraoral

There was a mild skeletal Class 3 dental base relationship and a reduced lower face height. There was no evidence of facial asymmetry nor could a displacement be detected on closure. The lips were competent.

Intraoral

General condition of the mouth
The patient had about average caries experience for a 10-year-old and the upper right second deciduous molar had been extracted. The oral hygiene was good.

The *lower incisors* were spaced and proclined.

The *lower canines* were unerupted but appeared to be well placed to do so.

The *lower buccal segments* were uncrowded but the lower left first molar had an early occlusal cavity in need of treatment.

The *upper incisors*: the central incisors were of average inclination or perhaps very slightly proclined. There was adequate space for the unerupted lateral incisors which were palpable buccally.

The *upper canines* were unerupted but palpable high up in the buccal sulcus.

The *upper buccal segments* were well aligned and adequate space remained for the upper right second premolar.

With the teeth in occlusion there was a marked Class 3 incisor relationship with an average and complete overbite and a reverse overjet of 2 mm. There was no displacement on closing but the upper centreline was displaced to the right. The molar occlusion was a half-unit Class II on the right but almost Class I on the left.

Radiographic

The orthopantomogram was rather poor but all teeth apart from the upper third molars were present and in good pre-eruptive positions.

Cephalometric

The cephalometric tracing confirmed a mild skeletal Class 3 dental base relationship (SNA 85.5, corrected ANB 1.5°) but showed that although the lower face height was below average, the facial proportions were within normal limits.

SN 11 years

HISTORY

Reason for attendance

The father was a hospital consultant and had asked for an opinion as the family lived close to the unit.

Dental history

The patient was a regular attender for routine dental treatment.

Medical history

There was no relevant medical history.

EXAMINATION

Extraoral

There was a Class 1 skeletal base relationship with an average Frankfort/mandibular planes angle. The lips were competent but slightly everted in form.

Intraoral

General condition of the mouth
The oral hygiene was only average but the caries rate was low.

The *lower incisors* were proclined and crowded with the lateral incisors displaced slightly lingually.

The *lower canines*: the lower left canine was distally inclined; the lower right was vertical. Both canines were crowded.

The *lower buccal segments* were acceptably aligned and very mildly crowded.

The *upper incisors* were proclined and crowded with the lateral incisors displaced slightly palatal to the line of the arch. Both upper central incisors were mildly mesiolabially rotated.

The *upper canines* were mesially inclined but the upper right canine had been displaced slightly buccally by the retained deciduous canine.

The *upper buccal segments* were well aligned.

With the teeth in occlusion there was a Class II division 1 incisor relationship with a 5 mm overjet on the central incisors and a reduced and incomplete overbite. On both sides the canines were a half-unit Class II but the molars were Class I.

Radiographic

All teeth were present on x-ray with the exception of the upper third molars. There was evidence of molar crowding.

Cephalometric

After due allowance is made for the low SNA angle (75°) a skeletal Class I dental base relationship was confirmed (ANB angle = 1.5°; corrected 4.5°). The maxillary/mandibular planes angle was 27.5°. There was much less upper incisor proclination than had been suggested by the clinical appearance (113.5° to MxP) but the lower incisors showed moderate proclination (99.5° to MdP).

EH 13 years 11 months

HISTORY

Reason for attendance

The patient had been referred because she and her mother were concerned about the appearance of the upper anterior teeth.

Dental history

The patient has been a regular dental attender with her general dental practitioner.

Medical history

There was no relevant medical history.

EXAMINATION

Extraoral

The patient had a mild Class 3 dental base relationship with an average Frankfort/maxillary planes angle. The lips were apart at rest but the upper lip covered the greater part of the upper incisors.

Intraoral

General condition of the mouth
The oral hygiene was good and there was an average caries experience.

The *lower incisors* were of average inclination to the mandibular plane and slightly crowded. The lower lateral incisors were slightly distally inclined.

The *lower canines* were vertical and slightly lingually displaced.

The *lower buccal segments* were slightly crowded with the lower left second premolar slightly lingually crowded and the lower right first molar also displaced lingually.

The *upper incisors* were of average inclination and crowded with the laterals palatally displaced.

The *upper canines* were mesially inclined and crowded, with the upper left almost completely excluded from the arch and overlying the lateral.

The *upper buccal segments*: the left segment was well aligned but the right showed mild crowding with the second premolar palatally displaced.

With the teeth in occlusion there was a reduced incisor overjet and overbite. The lateral incisors were in linguo-occlusion but with a 3 mm reversed overbite. There was a slight forward displacement on closing from an initial contact on these teeth. The molar occlusion was a half-unit Class II on the right and on the left. The premolars were in bilateral crossbite.

Radiographic

All teeth including the third molars were present on x-ray.

Cephalometric

The Class 3 skeletal pattern was confirmed. There was an ANB angle of $-1°$ (corrected $+1.5°$) and the maxillary/mandibular planes angle was average at 25°. The lower incisors were slightly retroclined but the uppers were of average inclination.

MB 12 years 10 months

HISTORY

Reason for attendance

The patient had been referred by his practitioner for orthodontic advice. Both parent and patient were only slightly concerned about the malocclusion.

Dental history

The patient was a regular dental attender.

Medical history

There was no relevant medical history.

Social history

Unfortunately the family lived 32 miles from the unit and travel was difficult since the family had no car.

EXAMINATION

Extraoral

There was a severe Class 2 skeletal pattern with average Frankfort/mandibular planes angle. The lips were incompetent with the lower lip trapped behind the upper incisors.

Intraoral

General condition of the mouth
The oral hygiene was only fair and there were extensive restorations in all four first permanent molars.

The *lower incisors* were proclined and well aligned.

The *lower canines* were slightly distally inclined but well aligned.

The *lower buccal segments*: the lower left first premolar was a microdont tooth.

The *upper incisors* were slightly proclined and spaced.

The *upper canines* were slightly distally inclined.

The *upper buccal segments* were well aligned.

With the teeth in occlusion there was a Class II division 1 incisor relationship with an overjet of 10 mm and overbite which was increased and complete on the palate. The molar occlusion was a full unit Class II on both sides.

Radiographic

The upper right third molar appeared to be absent and there was only slight evidence of the lower left third molar.

Cephalometric

There was a severe skeletal 2 pattern with a corrected ANB of 6° and an average maxillary/mandibular planes angle of 28.5°. Both the upper and the lower incisors were proclined (121° to MxP; 104.5° to MdP).

SR 12 years 8 months

HISTORY

Reason for attendance

The parents were concerned about the proclined upper lateral incisors.

Dental history

The patient had received regular dental treatment. The lower right second deciduous molar had been lost at 9 years of age.

Medical history

There was no relevant medical history.

EXAMINATION

Extraoral

The patient appeared to be skeletal Class 1 with an average face height and Frankfort/mandibular planes angle. The lips were competent and the lip line was about halfway up the labial surfaces of the upper central incisors.

Intraoral

General condition of the mouth
The patient was dentally rather late and was still in the late mixed dentition. The oral hygiene was good and the caries rate average.

The *lower incisors* were slightly retroclined and slightly crowded.

The *lower canines* were both distally inclined.

The *lower buccal segments*: the left was well aligned; the right was crowded with both premolars unerupted and short of space.

The *upper incisors*: the centrals were slightly retroclined but the laterals proclined and mesiolabially rotated in the classical Class II division 2 arrangement.

The *upper canines* were unerupted and could not be palpated.

The *upper buccal segments* were well aligned although the upper right second deciduous molar was still retained.

With the teeth in occlusion the incisor relationship was Class II division 2 with an overjet of 2 mm and an overbite which was increased and complete but just maintained tooth contact. The lower centreline was displaced to the right by 1.5 mm. The molars were Class I on the left and slightly Class III on the right.

Radiographic

All teeth were present including third molars. There appeared to be little sign of resorption of the upper right deciduous canine; parallax views confirmed that both the permanent canines, and particularly the right, were palatally misplaced.

Cephalometric

Tracing showed the patient to be within the range of skeletal 1 when the raised SNA of 85° is allowed for (corrected ANB of 3°). There was a slightly low maxillary/mandibular planes angle (23.5°). The lower incisors were of average angulation when the low maxillary/mandibular planes angle is allowed for and the upper central incisors were quite severely retroclined at 91.5° to the maxillary plane.

LM 12 years 1 month

HISTORY

Reason for attendance

The patient reattended for review, having originally been seen a year earlier at the request of her general dental practitioner.

Dental history

When first seen at 11 years 1 month, a number of deciduous teeth were retained and the upper right deciduous molar and the lower right second deciduous molars were showing signs of submergence. Six months later the upper molars had been shed but the lower had become more seriously submerged and was therefore removed under local anaesthesia.

Medical history

There was no relevant medical history.

EXAMINATION

Extraoral

The patient was thought to have a very mild skeletal Class 2 dental base relationship with an average face height. The lips were incompetent but habitually held together. The lower lip was just behind the upper incisor tips.

Intraoral

General condition of the mouth
The oral hygiene was good and the caries experience limited to an occlusal restoration in the upper left first molar.

The *lower incisors* were slightly proclined and well aligned.

The *lower canines* were upright and well aligned.

The *lower buccal segments* were slightly spaced and the teeth well aligned. The lower right second premolar had yet to erupt but had adequate space.

The *upper incisors* were proclined and generally well aligned, with the exception of the upper right lateral which had a slight mesiopalatal rotation.

The *upper canines* were mesially inclined and well aligned.

The *upper buccal segments* were well aligned.

With the teeth in occlusion there was a Class II division 1 incisor occlusion with an overjet of 9 mm and an overbite which was increased and complete (with tooth-to-tooth contact). The incisor centrelines were correct with each other and the midline of the face. The molar occlusion was a full unit Class II on the left and almost a full Class II unit on the right.

Radiographic

On the bimolars taken by the dental practitioner, both upper third molars and the lower left third molar were developing. The upper left first molar had a large restoration with evidence of some caries beneath it. (This was subsequently restored and considered to have a good prognosis.)

Cephalometric

The tracing confirmed the clinical impression. The sagittal jaw relationship just came within the Class 1 range with an ANB of 4° (SNA = 81.5°). The maxillary/mandibular angle was low but the lower face height was average at 61 mm. The upper incisors were markedly proclined at 126° to the maxillary plane, as were the lowers (109° to MdP) even after allowance is made for the reduced maxillary/mandibular planes angle.

ML 10 years 1 month

HISTORY

Reason for attendance

The patient attended the Primary Treatment Unit of the Dental School because her mother was concerned about the irregularity of her upper anterior teeth.

Dental history

Although nominally under the care of the Community Dental Service, ML appeared to have attended for little dental treatment apart from deciduous extractions. The patient was advised to seek routine dental care and subsequently decided to register with a local general dental practice.

EXAMINATION

Extraoral

There was a mild Class 2 skeletal pattern and a slightly reduced Frankfort/mandibular planes angle. The lips were competent and the lower lip, which was rather everted, rested halfway up the labial surfaces of the upper central incisors.

Intraoral

General condition of the mouth
The oral hygiene was good and by the time the patient began treatment she had a well cared for mouth, in the mixed dentition with good quality restorations in the first molars and some of the deciduous molars.

The *lower incisors* were of average inclination to the mandibular plane but crowded with the lower centreline to the left.

The *lower canines* were both distally inclined, the lower left being partially excluded from the arch and buccally displaced.

The *lower buccal segments* were slightly crowded on the right and more severely crowded on the left where the lower first premolar was impacted beneath the second deciduous molar.

The *upper incisors*: the central incisors were well aligned but retroclined. The upper lateral incisors were crowded and proclined with typical mesiolabial rotations.

The *upper canines* were unerupted and short of space but were palpable buccally and seemed to be slightly mesially inclined.

The *upper buccal segments* were well aligned on the left but slightly crowded on the right.

With the teeth in occlusion there was a Class II division 2 incisor occlusion with an overjet of 6.5 mm and an increased overbite which was just complete on the palate. Had they been present in the mouth the canines would have been a full unit Class II. The molar occlusion was a half-unit Class II on the left and a full unit Class II on the right.

Radiographic

All successional teeth and both lower third molars were present on x-ray and there were early signs of the crypt of the upper left third molar. The restorations in the first permanent molars appeared to be rather deep but sound.

Cephalometric

Assessment showed that there was a marked skeletal Class 2 dental base relationship with an ANB angle of 7° (corrected 6°) and a reduced maxillary/mandibular planes angle (19°). The upper incisors were markedly retroclined (98.5° to MxP) but the lower were only very slightly retroclined after allowance had been made for the low FM angle.

NO 14 years 4 months

HISTORY

Reason for attendance

The patient had originally been seen at the request of the Community Dental Service. At that time the patient complained that his front teeth 'did not bite together very well'.

Dental history

There was no history of trauma to the upper anterior teeth, neither was there a digit-sucking habit.

Medical history

There was no relevant medical history.

EXAMINATION

Extraoral

The patient appeared to have a near normal anteroposterior jaw relationship with an average lower face height. The lips were competent and the lower lip rested about halfway up the labial surfaces of the upper central incisors.

Intraoral

General condition of the mouth
The oral hygiene was good and the caries rate about average.

The *lower incisors* were slightly retroclined but well aligned apart from acceptable distolabial rotations of the central incisors.

The *lower canines* were upright and well aligned.

The *lower buccal segments* were well aligned.

The *upper incisors* were of average angulation. There was a median diastema and the upper left central was slightly mesiolabially rotated whilst the upper right showed a slight distolabial rotation which was accentuated by a distal angulation. The upper left lateral incisor had a marked mesiolabial rotation.

The *upper canines* were mesially inclined and well aligned with some space distal to both teeth.

The *upper buccal segments* were well aligned.

With the teeth in occlusion the incisor occlusion was on the borderline between Class I and Class II division 1. The overjet was 4.5 mm on the left central incisor and 7.5 mm on the right. The overbite was slightly increased but complete and the centrelines coincided.

The molar occlusion was Class I on the right but mildly Class III on the left.

Radiographic

All teeth including third molars were present and appeared to be of good prognosis.

Cephalometric

The skeletal Class 1 dental base relationship was confirmed. There was an SNA of 87° and an ANB angle of 5.5° (corrected at 2.5°). The lower face height and maxillary/mandibular planes angle (28°) were average. The upper incisors were ideally angulated in the sagittal plane at 110.5° to the maxillary plane but the lower incisors were 6° below the mean at 86.5° to the mandibular plane.

IR 13 years 7 months

HISTORY

Reason for attendance

The patient was referred by her dental officer in the Community Dental Service for advice about her upper incisor irregularity.

Dental history

The patient had been a regular attender at the local community clinic since she was 8 years old.

Medical history

There was no relevant medical history.

Social history

The family lived 5 miles away and had no car but there was a good local bus service.

EXAMINATION

Extraoral

The patient had a near normal dental base relationship. The Frankfort/mandibular planes angle appeared to be low (later shown to be untrue; see below under Cephalometric) although the lower face height was thought to be within normal limits. The lips were competent.

Intraoral

General condition of the mouth
The oral hygiene was good and the caries rate average for a 13 year old at that time.

The *lower incisors*: there were only three lower incisors which appeared to be of average inclination to the mandibular plane. It was not possible to deduce which tooth was absent but the remaining three were well aligned.

The *lower canines*: the lower right was well aligned, the left had an acceptable distolingual rotation. Both were mesially inclined and there was slight space distal to both teeth.

The *lower buccal segments* were well aligned.

The *upper incisors*: the central incisors were of average inclination and well aligned. The lateral incisors were crowded labially but without any associated rotation.

The *upper canines* were slightly mesially inclined and well aligned.

The *upper buccal segments* were well aligned.

With the teeth in occlusion there was a Class I incisor occlusion but with an increased overjet of 5 mm on the lateral incisors. The overbite was complete on the centrals but incomplete on the laterals. The upper centreline coincided with the middle of the central lower incisor. The buccal segments were an almost fully intercuspated Class I.

Radiographic

All third molars were developing.

Cephalometric

The patient had a skeletal 1 dental base relationship (ANB 2°; corrected 3°) with an average maxillary/mandibular planes angle. The lower incisors were slightly proclined but the upper incisors were slightly retroclined at 101.5° to the maxillary plane.

AT 11 years 10 months

HISTORY

Reason for attendance

The patient was referred by his general dental practitioner for orthodontic treatment.

Dental history

The patient had attended the family practice since the age of 3 years.

Medical history

There was no relevant medical history.

Social history

The patient was attending a private preparatory school and lived with his grandmother during the term time as his parents lived and worked abroad. He joined his parents during the holidays, which were usually taken abroad.

EXAMINATION

Extraoral

There was a near normal anteroposterior jaw relationship and the facial proportions were average. The lips were potentially competent with the upper incisors trapped outside the lower lip. Note that the facial photograph is not typical of the resting posture. The patient still sucked his right thumb.

Intraoral

General condition of the mouth
The oral hygiene was very poor and whilst the number of restorations was about average there was labial decalcification affecting all the upper incisors.

The *lower incisors* were slightly proclined and very slightly crowded.

The *lower canines*: the left was upright and the right slightly mesially inclined. Both were well aligned.

The *lower buccal segments* were well aligned, apart from the lower left first premolar which was slightly short of space and buccally displaced.

The *upper incisors* were proclined. There was a marked median diastema and a pronounced labial fraenum.

The *upper canines* were mesially inclined and well aligned with 1.5 mm space distal to each. The left deciduous canine was still present but very mobile.

The *upper buccal segments* were well aligned.

With the teeth in occlusion there was a marked Class II division 1 incisor occlusion. The overjet was 8.5 mm and the overbite average and incomplete. The buccal occlusion was Class I.

Radiographic

All teeth were present including the third molars.

Cephalometric

There was a Class 1 dental base relationship. The ANB angle was 5° (corrected 3.5°) The maxillary/mandibular planes angle was average (28°). The lower incisors were slightly proclined and the uppers almost 20° above the mean at 129° to the maxillary plane.

LJ 12 years 5 months

HISTORY

Reason for attendance

The patient had been referred by her general dental practitioner who had become concerned about the long-term effects of the very deep incisor overbite.

Dental history

The patient had always attended the family dental practice.

Medical history

There was no relevant medical history.

Social history

The patient attended a local public school as a weekly border. She was a keen musician and played the flute.

EXAMINATION

Extraoral

There was a moderate skeletal class 2 sagittal jaw relationship with a reduced lower face height and Frankfort/mandibular planes angle. The lips were competent with the lower rather everted in form.

Intraoral

General condition of the mouth
The oral hygiene was good and the caries experience average. All first molars were filled.

The *lower incisors* were of average angulation and well aligned.

The *lower canines* were distally inclined and well aligned with slight space behind them.

The *lower buccal segments* were well aligned.

The *upper incisors* were retroclined and crowded. The lateral incisors were slightly mesiolabially rotated, mesially inclined and rather small.

The *upper canines* were slightly mesially inclined and slightly distobuccally rotated. Here too there was a small amount of space distal to the canines.

The *upper buccal segments* were well aligned and there was slight space in the upper right second premolar site where the deciduous tooth had recently been exfoliated.

With the teeth in occlusion there was a typical Class II division 2 incisor relationship with an overjet of 3 mm and an overbite which was complete against the palate. There were no signs of trauma. The buccal segments were a full unit Class II.

Radiographic

Only the upper third molars showed signs of developing.

Cephalometric

The skeletal Class 2 pattern was confirmed by an ANB angle of 8° (corrected 6°). The lower face height was reduced, as was the maxillary/mandibular planes angle (21°) although the facial proportions were average. The lower incisors were at average inclination for a maxillary/mandibular planes angle of 21° but the upper incisors were markedly retroclined at 87° to the maxillary plane.

JS 12 years 6 months

HISTORY

Reason for attendance

The patient was referred by a local Community Dental Officer for advice about the severely increased overjet.

Dental history

The patient had been seen by the Community Dental Service since the age of 8 years, although she was not a particularly regular attender.

Medical history

There was no relevant medical history.

EXAMINATION

Extraoral

The patient had what appeared to be a marked skeletal Class 2 dental base relationship. The lower face height and Frankfort/mandibular planes angle appeared to be average but the lips were incompetent and were habitually apart most of the time. The lower lip looked as if it would just control the upper incisor at rest if these teeth were retracted.

Intraoral

General condition of the mouth
The oral hygiene was fair and the caries rate average.

The *lower incisors* were slightly proclined and slightly crowded with the lower left central incisor showing a very slight mesiolabial rotation.

The *lower canines* were both slightly mesially inclined and well aligned.

The *lower buccal segments* were well aligned.

The *upper incisors* were markedly proclined and spaced.

The *upper canines* were slightly mesially inclined and spaced.

The *upper buccal segments*: there was slight spacing between the premolars.

With the teeth in occlusion there was a severe Class II division 1 incisor occlusion. The overjet was 11.5 mm and the overbite increased and complete on the palate. However there was no sign of trauma and the upper and lower centrelines were coincident. The buccal occlusion was approaching Class I on both sides.

Radiographic

All second and third molars were of good size and developing normally with no sign of posterior crowding.

Cephalometric

There was a skeletal Class 2 base with an ANB angle of 8° (corrected 6°). The maxillary/ mandibular planes angle was average, as was the lower face height. The lower incisors proclined by about 5° above the mean at 97.5° to the mandibular plane but the upper were almost 20° proclined (129.5° to MxP).

SECTION FOUR

Treatment

This section comments frankly on the treatment carried out. In retrospect not all treatment plans were correct; even when they were, not all went entirely according to plan.

Cases key

JB 13 years 4 months

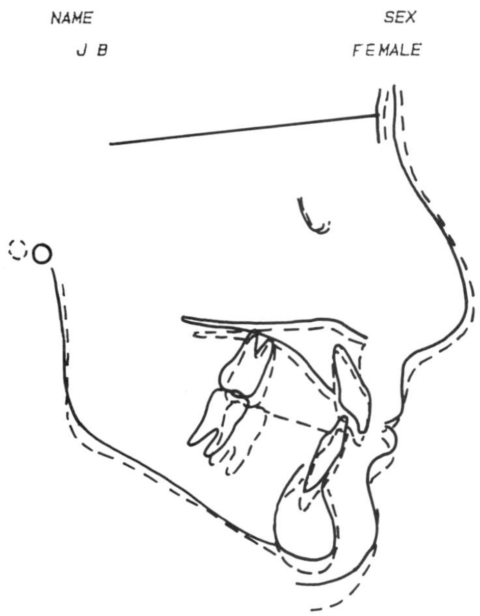

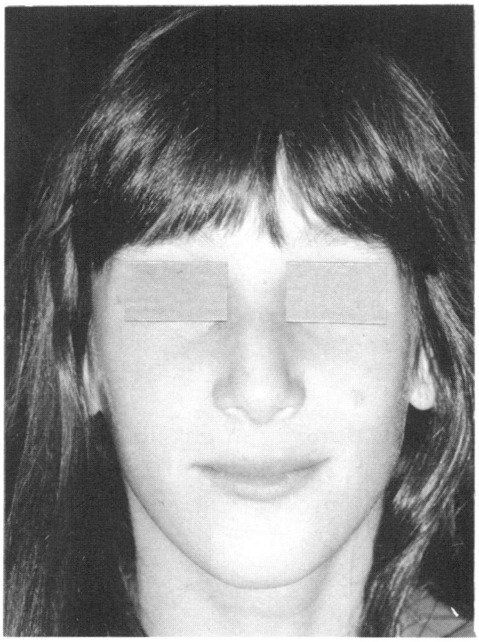

TREATMENT PLAN

Treatment aims

It was decided that the lower arch alignment at the time of presentation was acceptable but that there was evidence of molar crowding in the second and third molar regions. In the upper arch there was lack of space for the upper right canine and upper right lateral incisor. In this arch too there was evidence of molar crowding in the form of second and third molar 'stacking'. Aims were therefore:

1 Accommodation of the upper right canine and lateral incisor.
2 Relief of posterior crowding and preservation of the lower arch alignment.
3 Correction of the buccal occlusion on the right.

Treatment means

Loss of lower second molars (unlike the loss of the third molar) has been shown to reduce the tendency of lower incisor crowding to worsen during late adolescence. In view of this and as the lower third molars were favourably placed, the lower second molars were removed. These teeth were also considered the appropriate choice in the upper arch where their loss would facilitate the distal movement of both upper buccal segments but particularly the right.

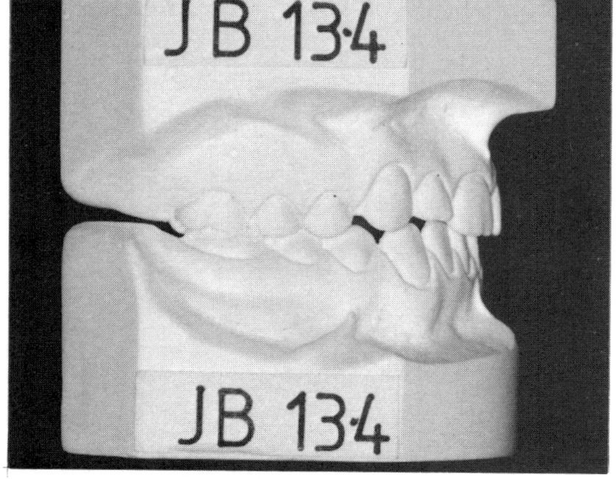

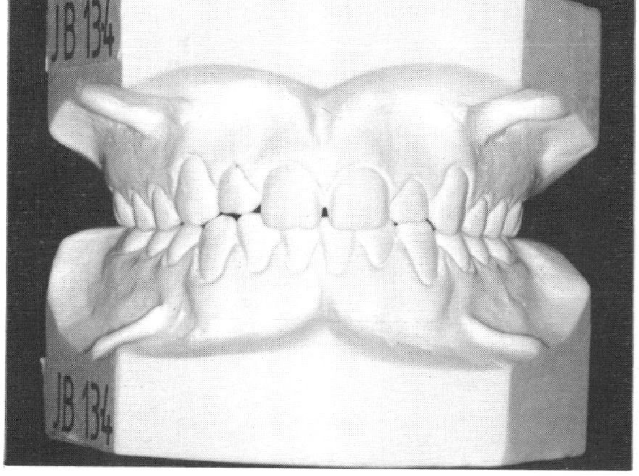

Appliance design

Because both the right canine and lateral incisor were favourably inclined, removable appliances could be used. The first appliance was an upper screw plate. No provision was made for headgear since one buccal segment can be retracted without extraoral support to the anchorage if the second molar has been removed. (It would however have been a simple matter to add molar tubes should this optimism have proved to be misplaced!)

A second appliance was then required to tip the canine buccally and retrocline the lateral incisor. For buccal movement in the premolar and molar region the shape of the plate makes the T-spring the obvious choice (if one attempts to use a Z-spring the bulk of the appliance will be unnecessarily increased). For the same reason the Z-spring is to be preferred at the front of the mouth. However in the canine region it is possible to use either a Z-spring or a T-spring.

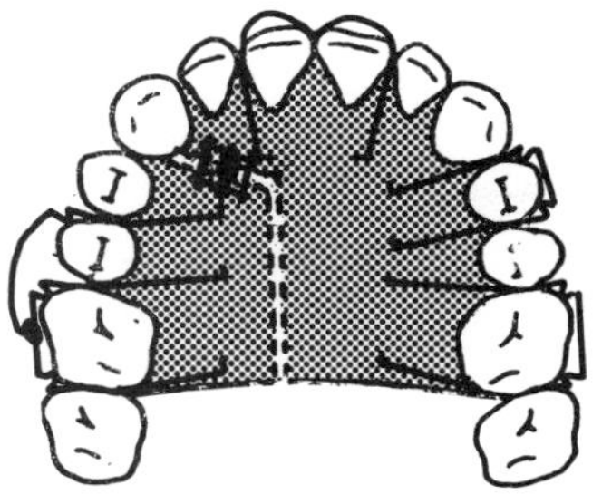

Appliance 1

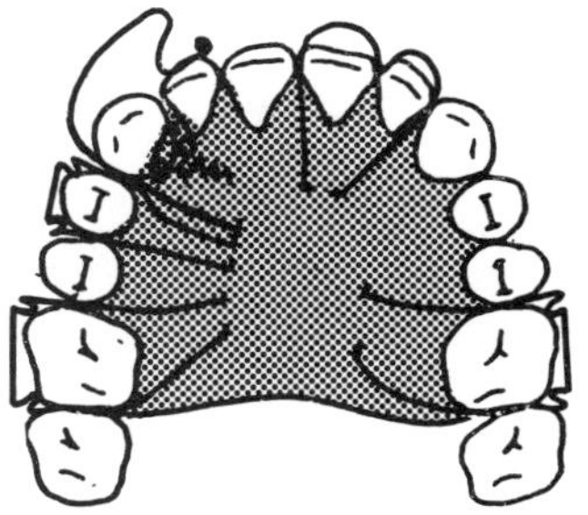

Appliance 2

COMMENTS ON TREATMENT

Treatment took 12 months and was followed by 6 months' retention (3 months full time and 3 months nights only wear). The models are shown 18 months out of retention. Radiographically the lower third molars (which are much less predictable after the loss of the second molars than those in the upper arch) appear to be in excellent position to erupt and indeed did so by the age of 16 years.

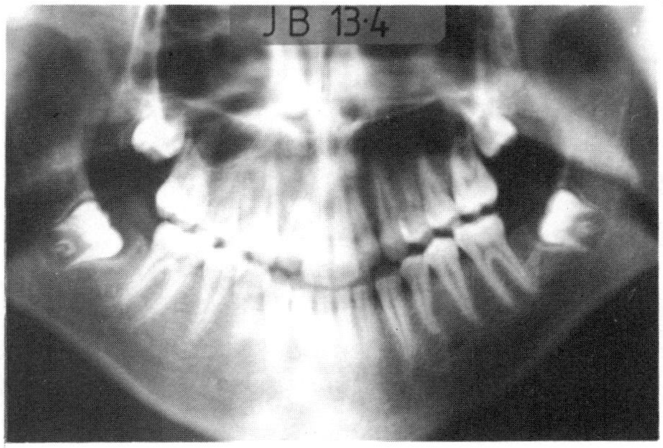

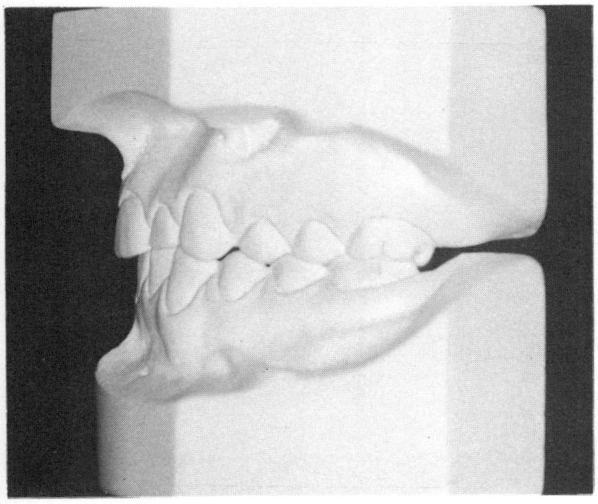

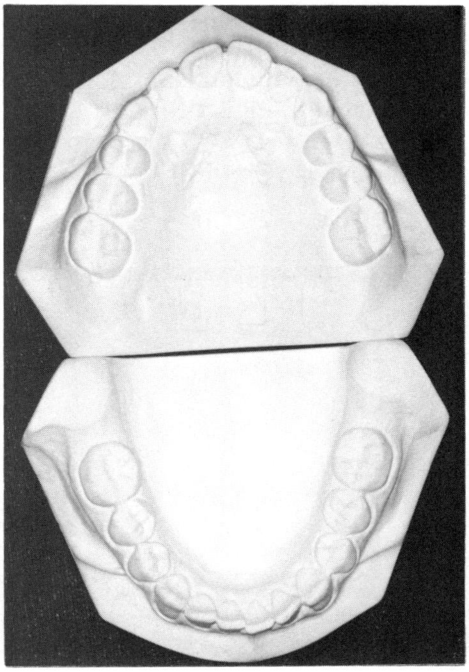

LB 36 years 4 months

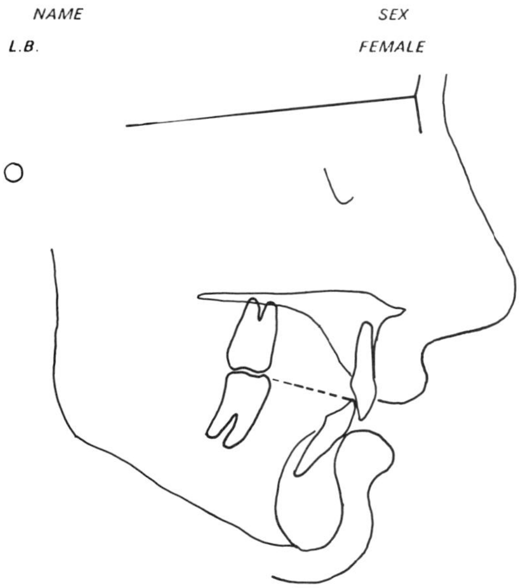

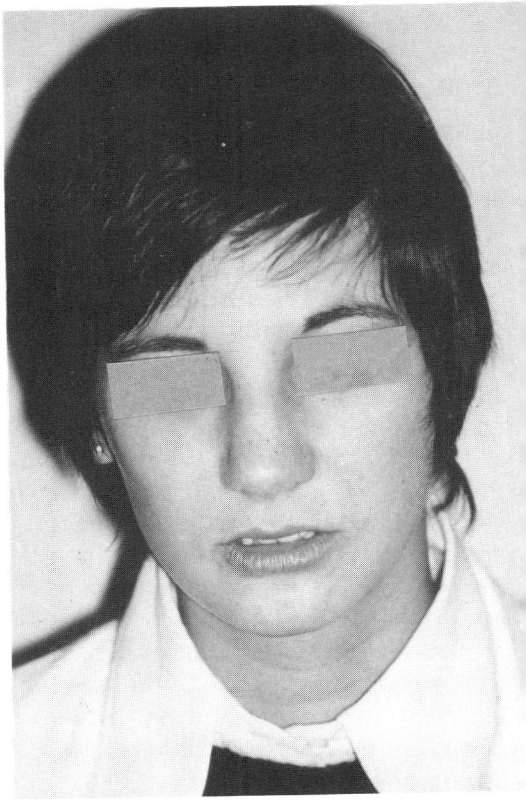

TREATMENT PLAN

Treatment aims

These were:

1 To intrude the lower right second molar.
2 Then to move the upper second molar back into a correct articulation with its opponent.

This would allow a bridge to be made to replace the missing first molar. (The lower arch alignment and the incisor occlusion were considered acceptable although it was realized that the right first molar would eventually require a full gold crown.)

Treatment means

As the upper second molar was very mesially inclined it was felt that this could be tipped distally with a removable appliance. Although this would only partially correct the rotation, any occlusal shortcomings could be solved by modifiying the form of the gold crown required in the bridge construction. The overerupted second molar could be intruded initially by means of a local bite plane.

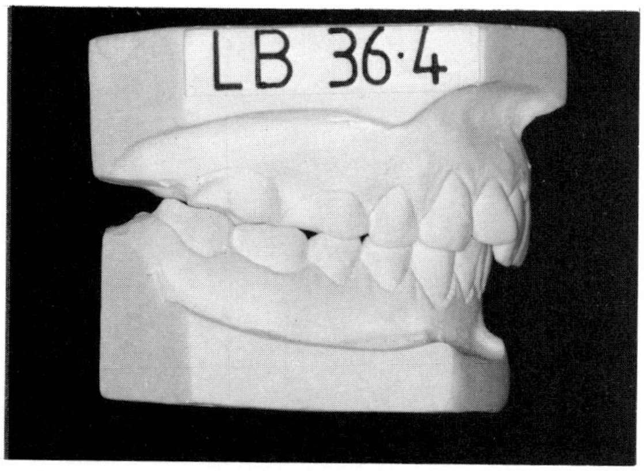

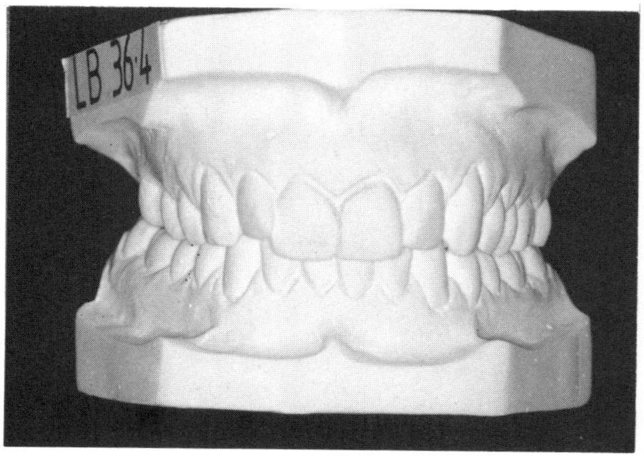

Appliance design

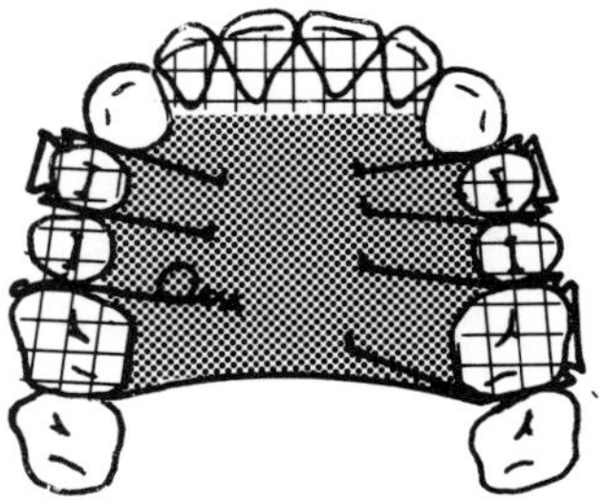

The retraction of the molar was performed by a palatal spring in 0.6 mm wire – the usual diameter for molar movement. It will be noted that there are both anterior and posterior bite planes. This was to allow the molar movement to begin at once (i.e. before the lower molar had been fully intruded) without risking an increase in the incisor overbite. Acrylic was removed occlusally and distally to the upper second molar to ensure that the tooth was free to move. The patient carried out her own adjustment by gradually reducing the left posterior and anterior planes until the lower second molar was level with the occlusal plane.

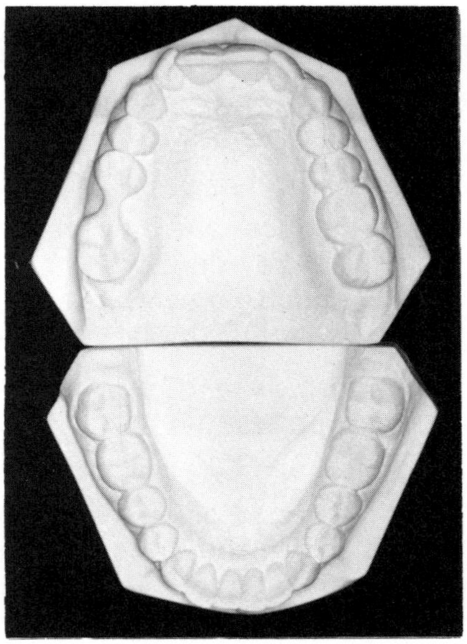

COMMENTS ON TREATMENT

Treatment proceeded uneventfully and was complete in only 3 months. The occlusion is shown 15 years after the fitting of the bridge which took place immediately before the appliance was discarded.

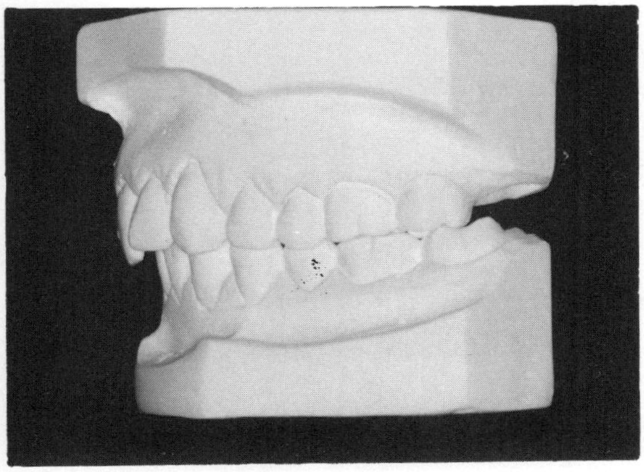

CB 14 years 8 months

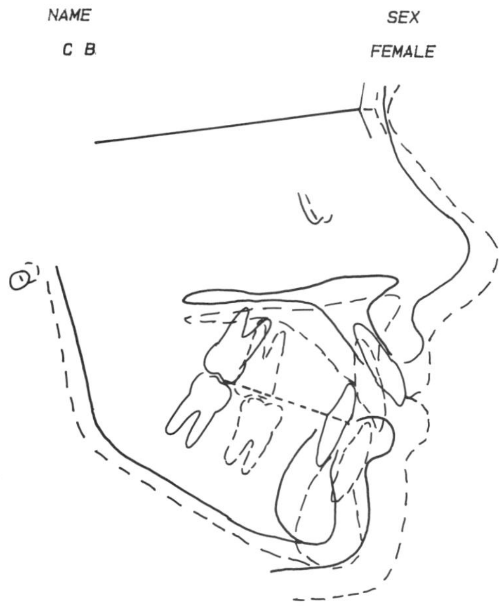

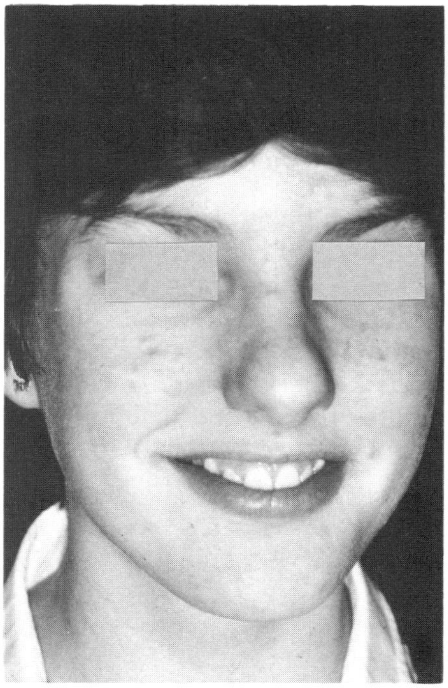

TREATMENT PLAN

Treatment aims

These were:

1 To reduce and relieve the incisor and canine crowding.
2 To reduce the overbite and overjet.
3 To correct the molar occlusion.

Treatment means

Even with the loss of one premolar per quadrant it was anticipated that anchorage might be a problem. In the upper arch all the premolar space would be required for relief of crowding and the reduction of the overjet. In the lower arch almost a full premolar unit was required to relieve crowding in the left quadrant. Care would be needed to avoid any further increase in the lower face height which would worsen the lip incompetence and aggravate the sagittal discrepancy.

Although the upper incisors were proclined, the greatly increased overjet (and underlying skeletal discrepancy) meant that simple tipping of these teeth would cause them to become severely retroclined during full overjet correction. Fixed appliances were therefore indicated to effect 'apical control' during incisor retraction. The unfavourable angulation of the lower canines meant that a fixed appliance would be required in the lower arch also (i.e. spontaneous alignment or uprighting could not be anticipated following extraction and in any case there was no excess space to allow uncontrolled space closure to take place). For all these reasons full upper and lower fixed

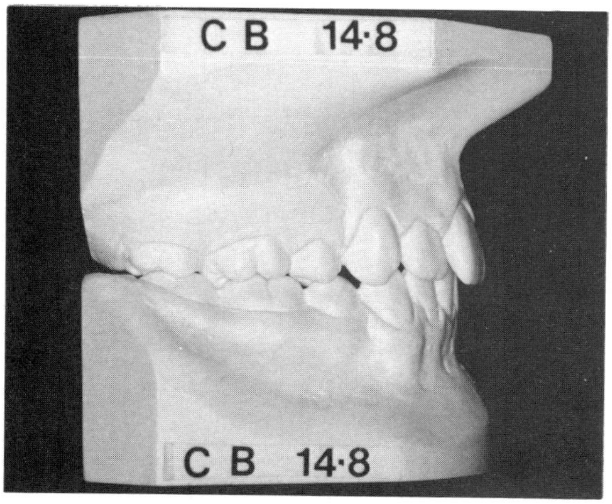

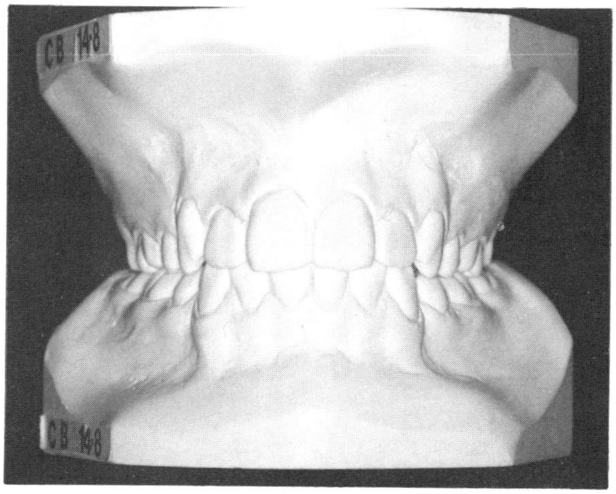

appliances were felt to be obligatory and this was classified as a moderately difficult case.

As the patient was keen to begin treatment and there was some reason for believing that the upper incisors were at risk from accidental damage (which reaches a peak incidence at this age) it was felt that treatment should begin as soon as possible. Because conventional fixed appliance treatment would have to be delayed until the premolars had erupted, it was decided to undertake an initial course of treatment using a functional appliance of the Harvold activator type.

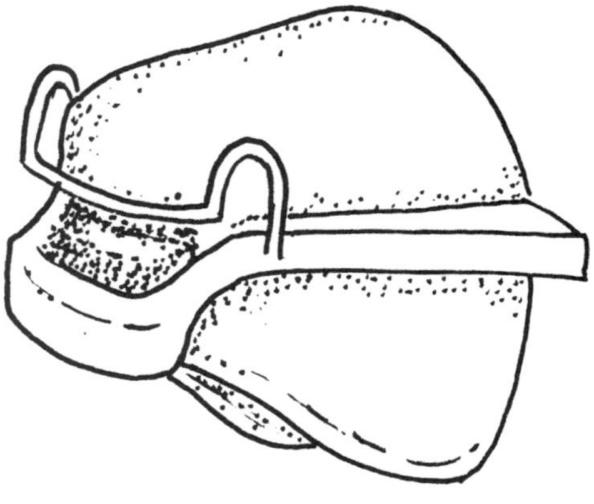

COMMENTS ON TREATMENT

The activator succeeded in reducing the overjet by 4 mm. Begg fixed appliance treatment including the loss of all first premolars began at 11 years and lasted just over a year. Unfortunately, shortly after the retainers were discarded, the patient entered a period of rapid growth and the overjet started to relapse. The use of a new activator for a short period reattained full overjet reduction and retention was continued with this appliance until the patient ceased growth in stature at 14½ years. Although now stable 2 years out of retention, the patient has a rather 'gummy' smile. Fortunately this does not concern her but on reflection rather more intrusive mechanics could have been employed and might have improved matters. Interestingly, during treatment the growth pattern was almost purely horizontal and it was only during the retention period that the lower face height showed a significant increase. Hence it seems unlikely that the mechanics of treatment worsened the inherent problems of the case.

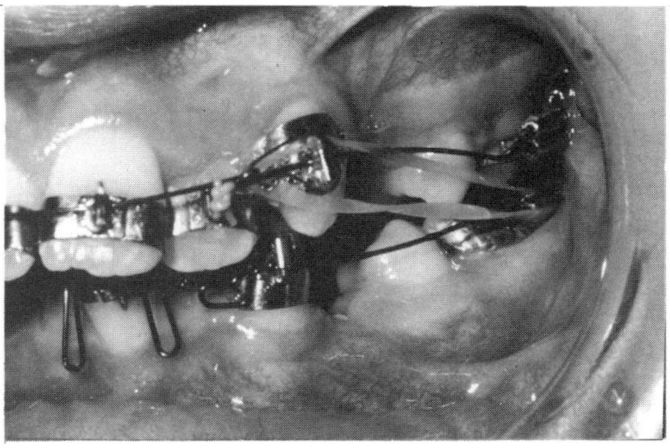

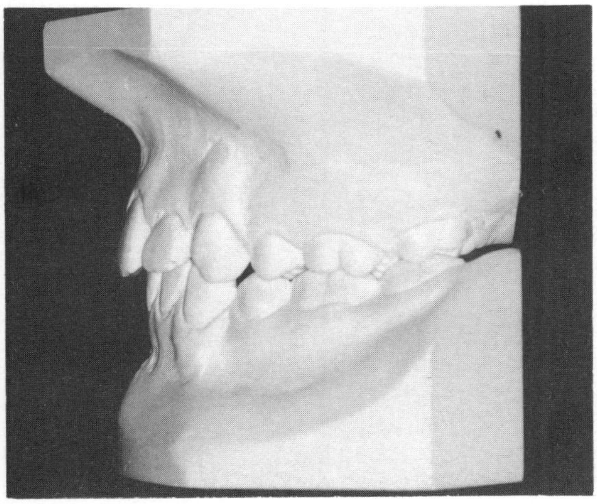

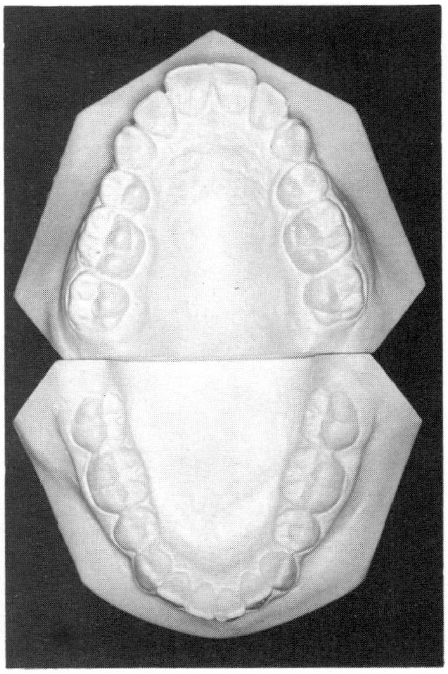

AT 18 years 10 months

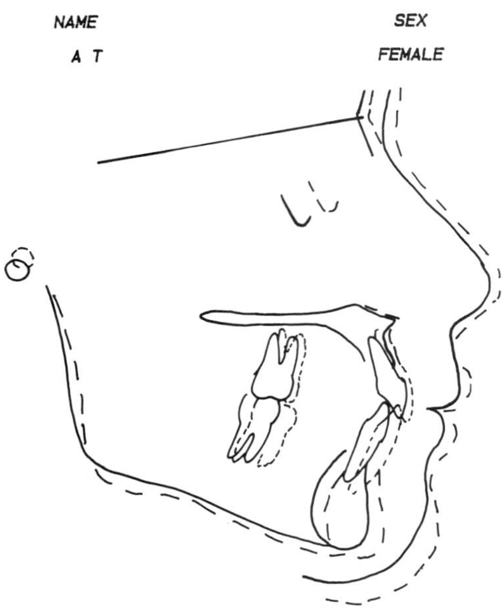

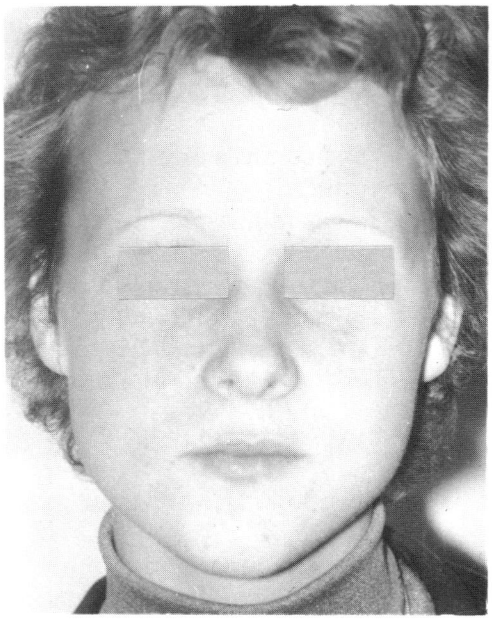

TREATMENT PLAN

Treatment aims

1 To relieve the upper and lower incisor crowding.
2 To align the upper and lower incisors.
3 To correct the premolar crossbite.

(As the logical choice was to remove the supplemental it follows that a further treatment aim will be to correct the molar occlusion.)

Treatment means

It was felt that there was insufficient crowding to justify extraction of premolar teeth once the lower supplemental had been removed but it was recognized that this would still leave unresolved posterior crowding. Although it was impossible to determine which was the additional lower incisor, the choice for extraction clearly lay with the middle incisor because it was flanked with distally inclined teeth which could then be expected to upright to some extent by tipping towards the extraction space.

There was evidence of moderate posterior crowding. In the upper arch, removal of second molars was indicated as this would permit a small amount of distal movement to be obtained for alignment of the upper labial segment using headgear to distalize the upper buccal segments. As always, there was some debate as to whether second or third molars should be removed in the lower arch. On the left the matter was settled by the condition of the lower second molar. On the right it was decided to remove the third molar because of the unpredictable behaviour of the lower third molar following loss of the second molar. Fixed appliances were thought to be required to align fully the lower and upper labial segments but the patient adamantly refused this part of the treatment.

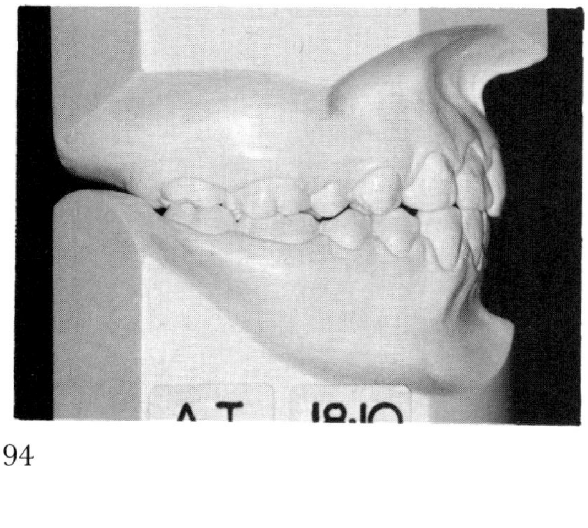

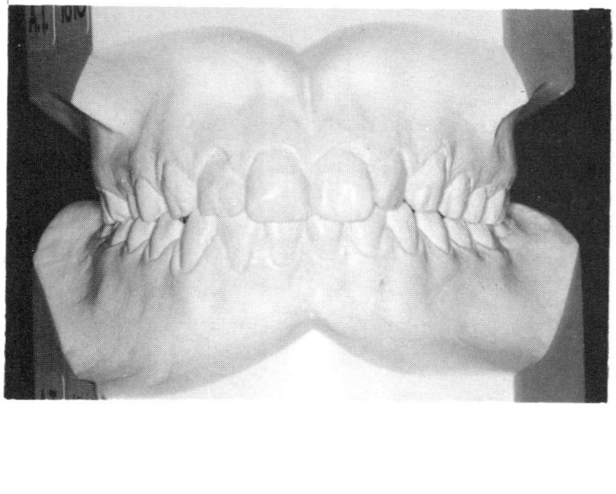

Appliance design

Because we were hopeful that the patient would eventually accept a fixed appliance, it was decided to use molar bands for headgear attachment. (This avoids problems when the time comes to change to a full upper fixed appliance.) Once the molar occlusion had been corrected (partly by distal movement in the upper arch and partly by mesial migration in the lower arch caused by the removal of the supplemental), a removable appliance was fitted over the molar bands, as shown. Palatal springs were used to retract the first premolars and canines (as is usually the case, the second premolar followed the molar distally and required no additional retraction). The retention was provided posteriorly by clips around the molar tubes (0.8 mm) and anteriorly by a crib embracing the upper central incisors.

Following a further refusal by the patient to accept a fixed appliance a second removable appliance was fitted and a T-spring was applied to move the upper right second premolar buccally and a buccal spring to align the upper left lateral as far as possible.

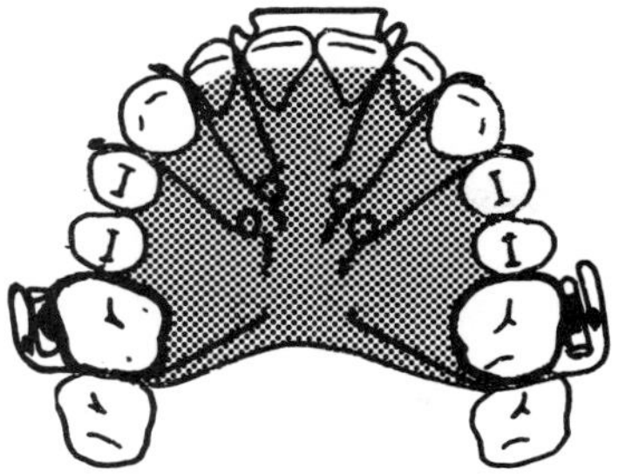

Appliance 1

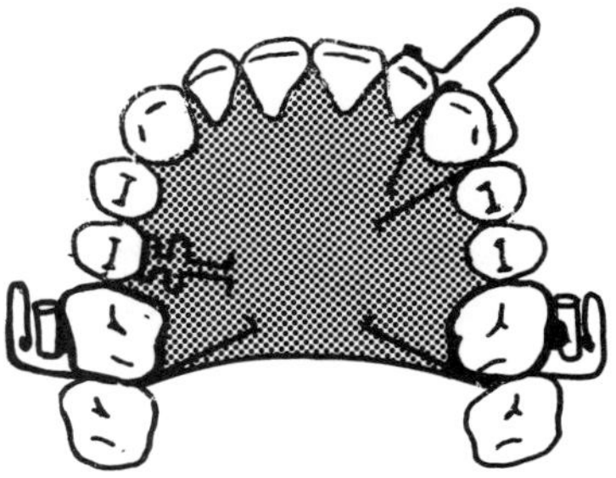

Appliance 2

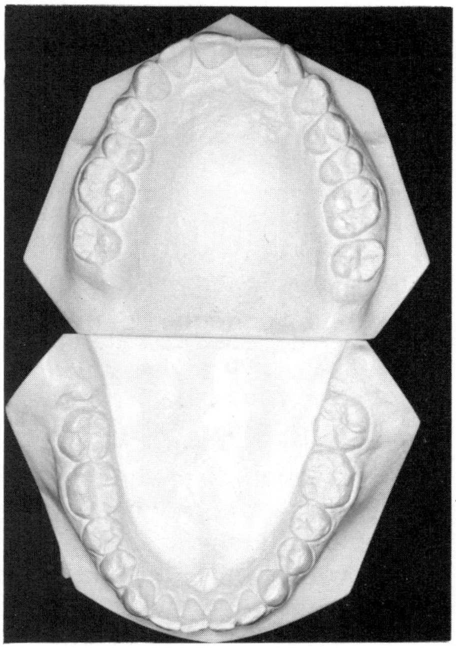

COMMENTS ON TREATMENT

The alignment in the lower arch was truly remarkable although it has to be said that this usually seems to be the case when a supplemental is removed in the lower incisor region. It is sad that the patient could not be persuaded to have an upper fixed appliance and the result here is a little disappointing. The lower left third molar can be seen to have erupted into an excellent position and the lower right was eventually removed surgically under local anaesthesia. In view of the extensive restoration in the right second molar it could be argued that it might have been better to have removed both lower second molars at the outset.

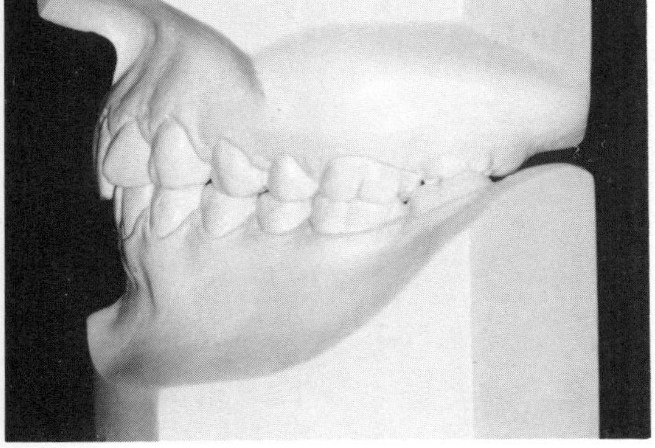

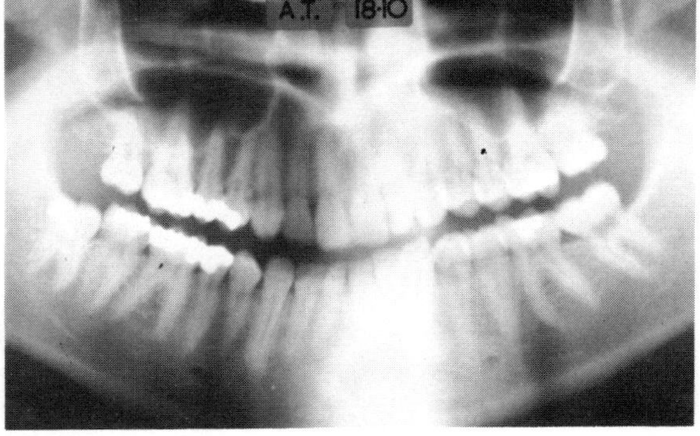

CW 24 years 9 months

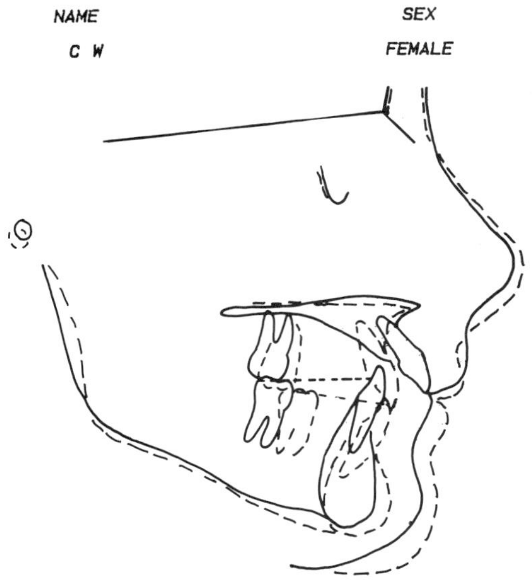

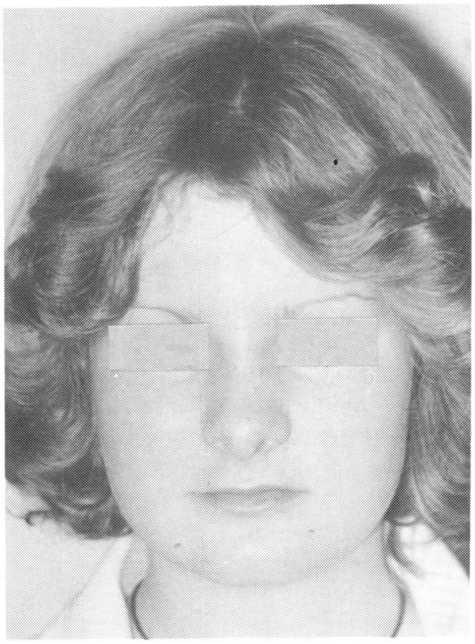

TREATMENT PLAN

Treatment aims

These were:

1 Elimination of the traumatic overbite.
2 Reduction of the overjet.
3 Relief of the crowding.
4 Alignment of the teeth within each arch including correction of the local crossbites.

Treatment means

The lower arch is sufficiently crowded to require extraction of premolars. There might be some argument as to whether these should be lower first or lower second premolars but the latter would only be acceptable if fixed appliances were to be used to ensure that the first premolar and first molar establish a good relationship to each other (see below). In the upper arch examination of the canine relationship demonstrates that a full premolar unit is required to enable the canines to achieve Class I. In other words there is no space to allow anchorage loss to occur. Hence the more teeth in the anchorage the better and reinforcement will be necessary either with headgear or by means of intermaxillary traction. The choice of extraction logically becomes one of first premolars in the upper arch, to give the maximum space for anterior retraction, and the need to preserve the present good molar occlusion dictates the loss of the first premolars in the lower arch also (rule 2). It also follows that since there will be some excess space in the lower arch, intermaxillary anchorage rather than extraoral anchorage is preferred.

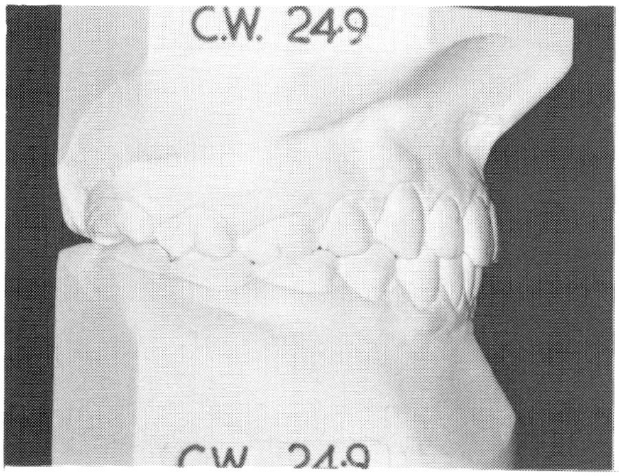

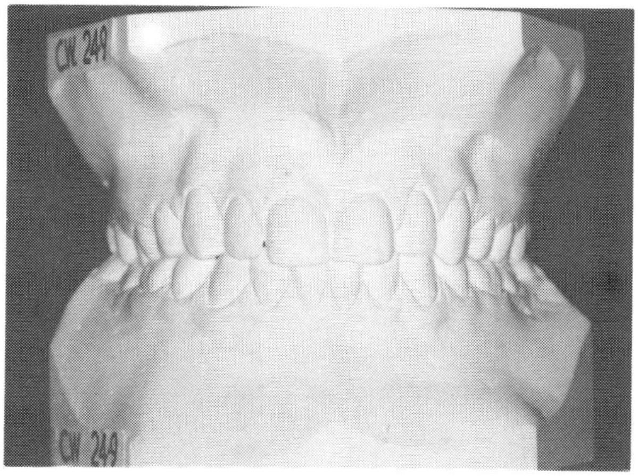

Appliance design

Fixed appliances are indicated on three grounds:

1 To enable a good incisor relationship to be obtained – with tooth to tooth contact and without excessive retroclination of the upper incisors.
2 To correct the rotation of the lower left canine.
3 To establish an acceptable angulation between the lower canines and second premolars.
4 To close up excess space in the lower arch.

COMMENTS ON TREATMENT

The case was treated with the Begg technique although any multibanded fixed appliance technique would have sufficed here. Perhaps the Begg technique is particularly suited to the reduction of deep overbite and in this case it also gave the opportunity to use the excess space in the lower arch in the reinforcement of upper arch anchorage through the use of Class II intraoral elastic traction.

Treatment took 2 years 5 months to complete and was followed by the usual 6-month period of retention with removable retainers. It will be noted that the lower incisors have become significantly proclined. This was unintentional and was caused by a damaged archwire late in the treatment (which also prolonged treatment time). Fortunately the teeth remained just on APo line and have remained stable in this position. Models are shown 10 years out of retention.

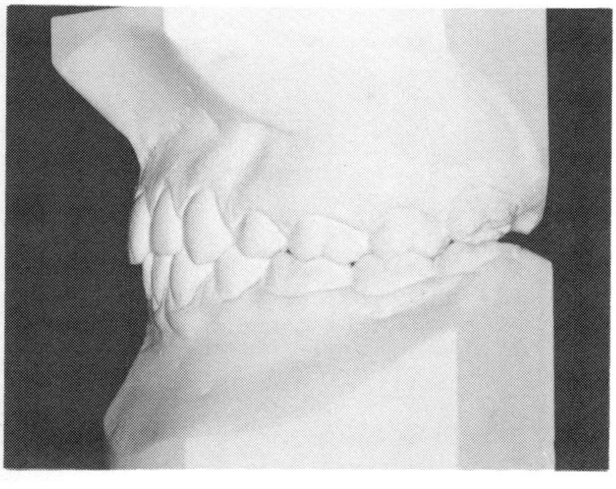

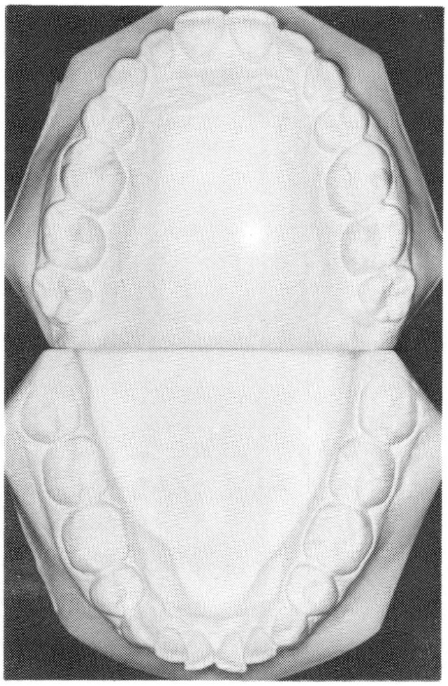

RP 15 years 3 months

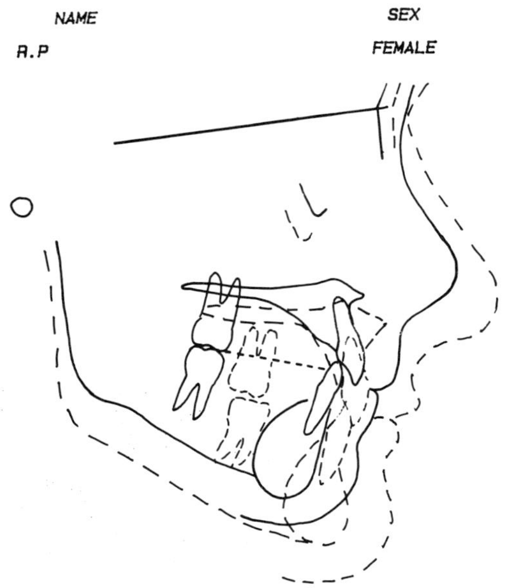

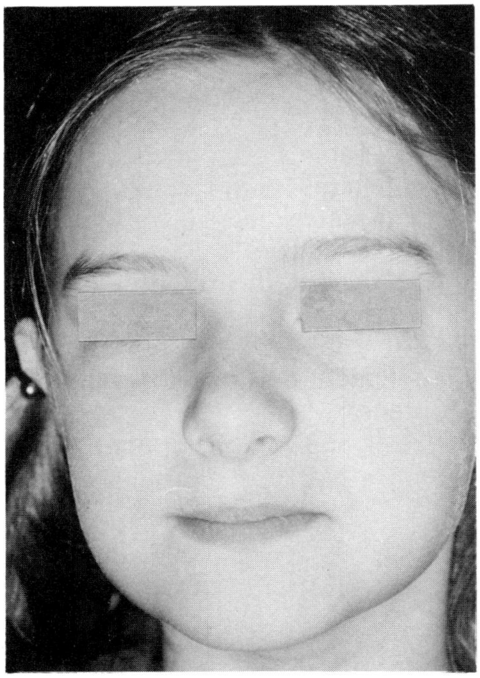

TREATMENT PLAN

Treatment aims

The incisor relationship is very acceptable and so the aims of treatment were:

1 To relieve crowding.
2 To advance the upper left lateral over the bite if necessary.

Treatment means

There was thought to be sufficient crowding in the canine region to justify loss of all four first premolars and it was believed that there would be favourable spontaneous changes following this. The molar occlusion was reasonably close to Class I and since both lower second deciduous molars had yet to be shed, the lower teeth might be expected to slide into a good Class I occlusion when this occurred. It seemed likely that an upper space-maintainer would eventually be required which could also be used to advance the upper left lateral over the bite. Initially though, spontaneous tooth movement would be observed whilst at the same time space closure would be closely monitored.

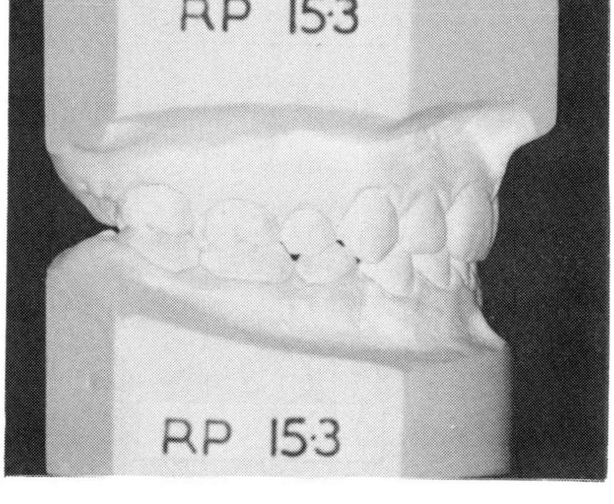

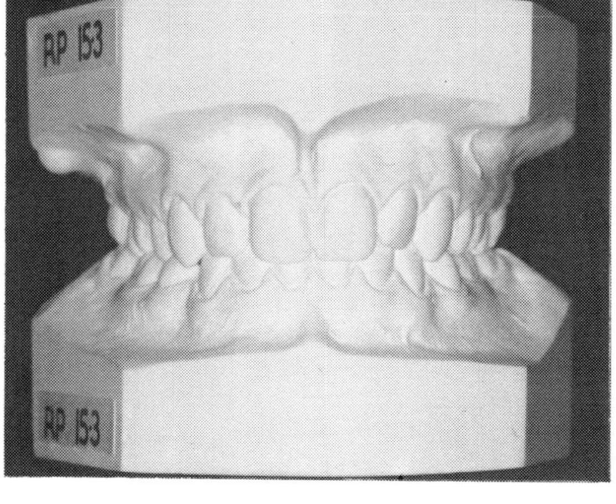

COMMENTS ON TREATMENT

In the event no active treatment and no space maintenance was required. Rather surprisingly, the lower left canine moved distally around the back of the upper lateral incisor and then moved mesially again in its correct bucco-lingual relationship. Restrictions of space preclude the inclusion of this interesting series of photographs.

Space closure was unexpectedly slow in the lower right quadrant, perhaps associated with the late appearance of the lower right third molar. When the crypt of this tooth finally appeared half the premolar space still remained but this subsequently closed rapidly. Altogether an excellent occlusion has been obtained by spontaneous tooth movement. The only point of criticism might be the slightly less than ideal angulation between the lower canine and second premolar.

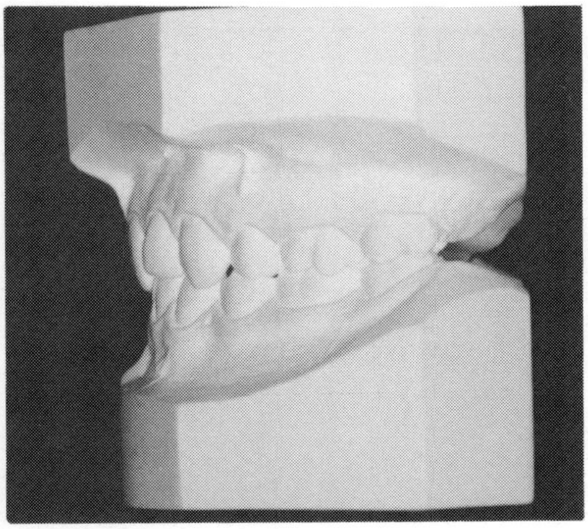

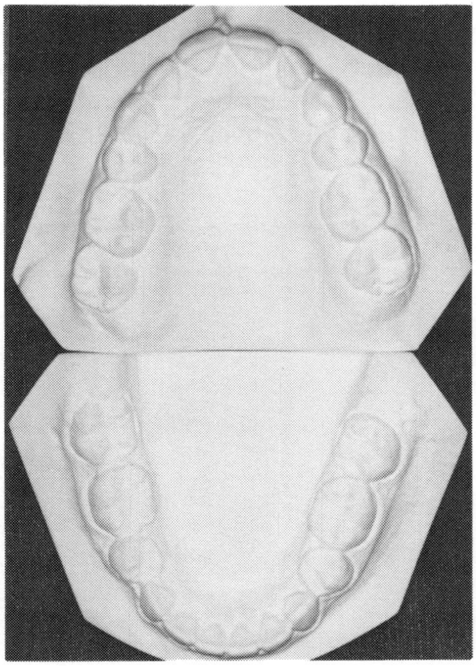

SD 22 years 3 months

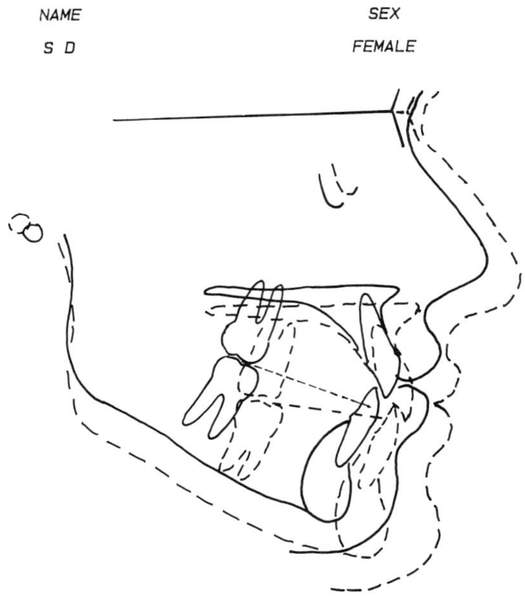

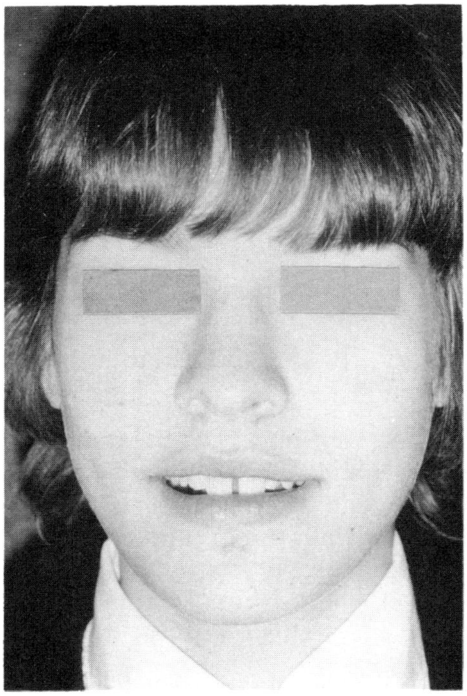

TREATMENT PLAN

Treatment aims

As there was clearly generalized spacing and a Class I incisor relationship, treatment was concerned only with alignment within the arches. There seemed little point in attempting to close the space in either arch. Treatment aims were therefore confined to:

1. Correcting the incisor crossbite and eliminating the mandibular displacement.
2. Derotation of both lateral incisors using some of the space available in the midline.

Treatment means

The rotation of the upper laterals dictated the use of a simple fixed appliance and edgewise technique was employed in the upper arch.

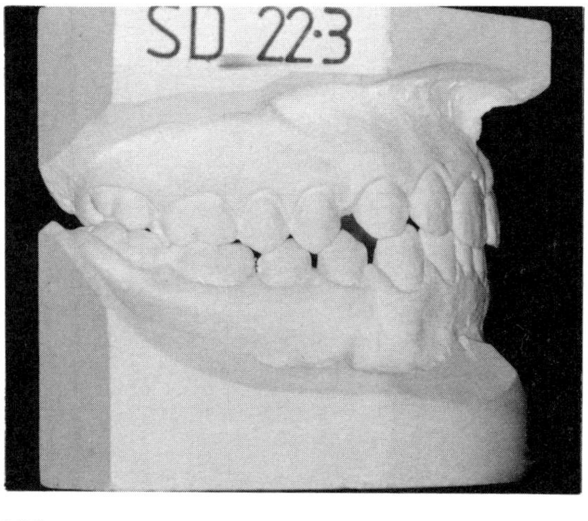

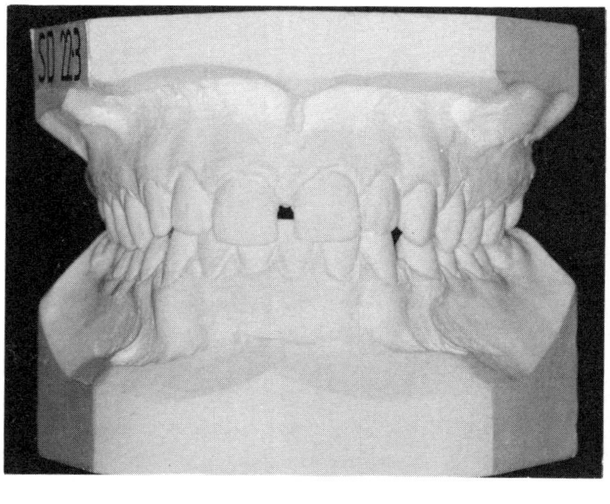

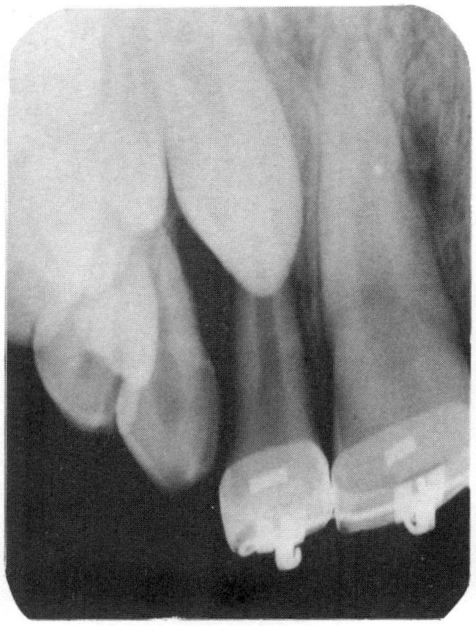

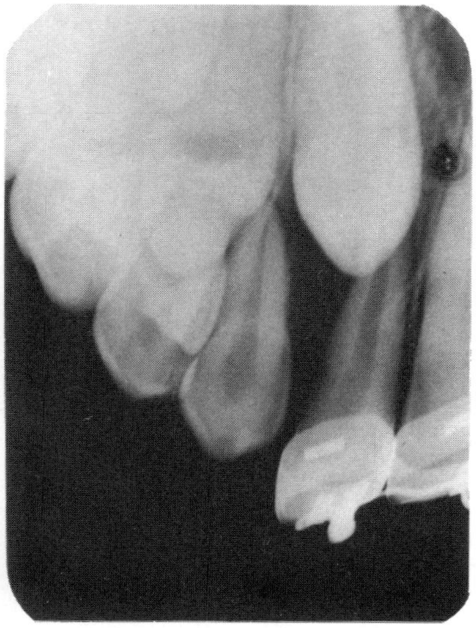

COMMENTS ON TREATMENT

The upper lateral incisors were aligned and overcorrected in 6 months. The teeth were pericised and then retained. At this time the right canine was still unerupted and could not be palpated; new films revealed it was becoming more displaced. (This is surprising in view of the fact that it is the upper right which appears to be most displaced on the pretreatment radiograph.) As the molar relationship was still Class II on the right (loss of the displacement to the left had only marginally improved this but had caused those on the left to become slightly Class II), headgear was applied to molar bands to distalize the molars and act as a space-maintainer, allowing both upper deciduous canines to be removed.

The justification for these extractions was that the loss of the upper right would encourage the permanent successor to align whilst the left would act as a balancing extraction. In fact, in view of the advanced resorption of this tooth it would have been lost very soon in any case and its extraction was probably unnecessary. No compensatory extractions were thought to be required in the lower arch, which had developed considerable space mesial to the canines.

At this point in the treatment the fixed appliance was removed but a sectional retainer was employed, tied in on the incisor brackets only. Six months later both upper canines had erupted. These teeth were found to be unusually small and only very slightly larger than the deciduous precursors. Records are shown just under 10 years out of all retention.

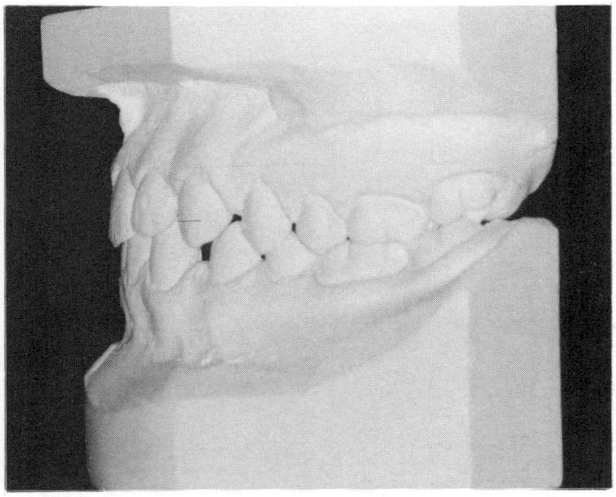

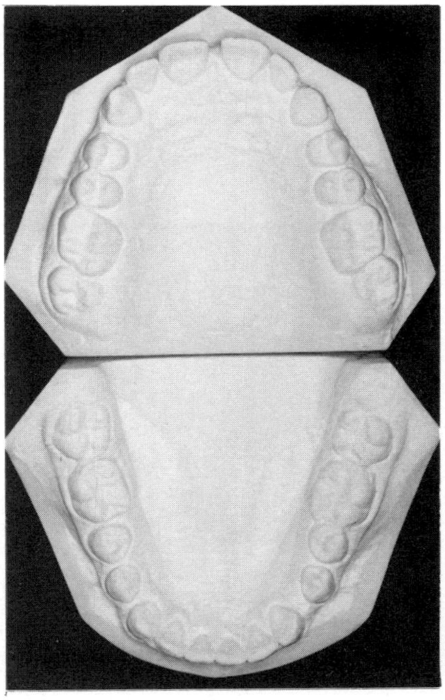

JK 14 years 6 months

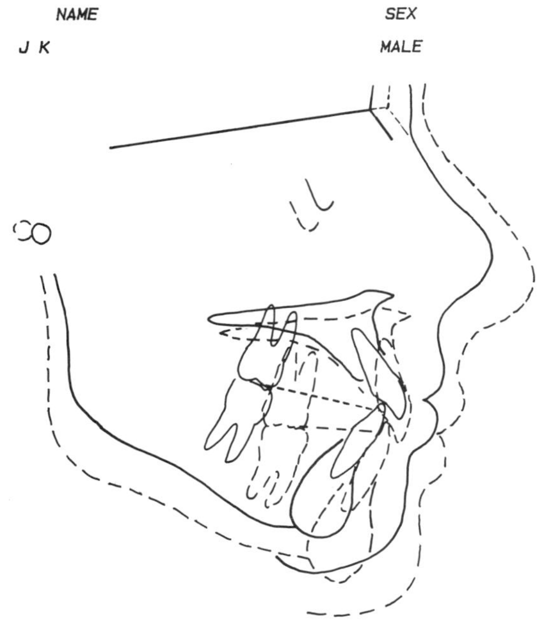

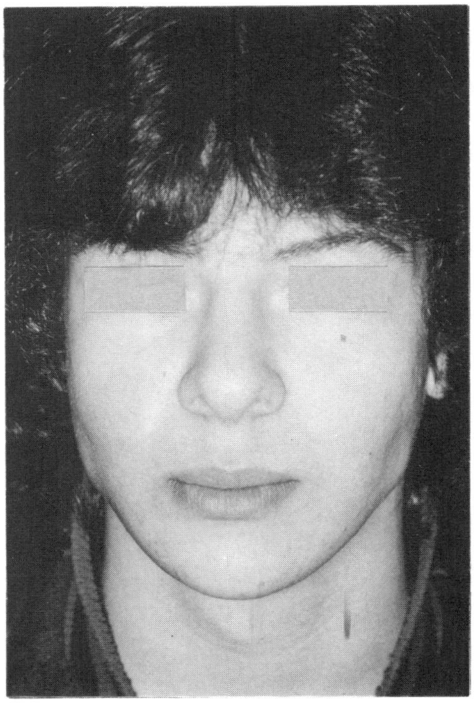

TREATMENT PLAN

Treatment aims

These were:

1 To relieve crowding.
2 Reduce the overbite and overjet.
3 To maintain the Class I molar relationship.

Treatment means

There was thought to be sufficient crowding to justify the loss of all four first premolars. In the lower arch it was anticipated that since the lower incisor crowding was confined to labio-lingual displacement, these would align spontaneously following premolar extraction. The favourable angulation of the upper canines and the fact that their rotations were acceptable suggested that the upper arch could be adequately treated by means of a removable appliance.

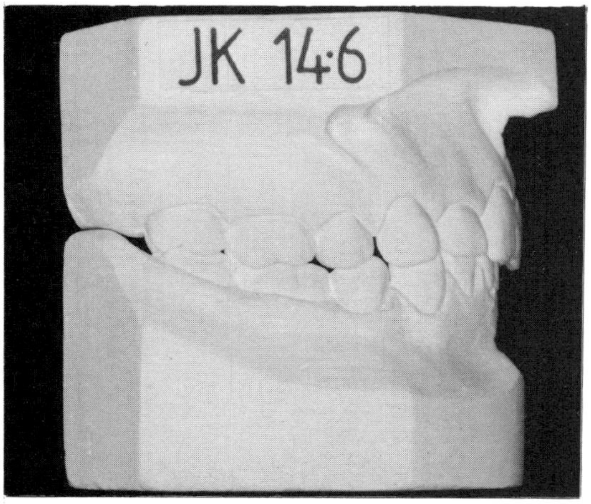

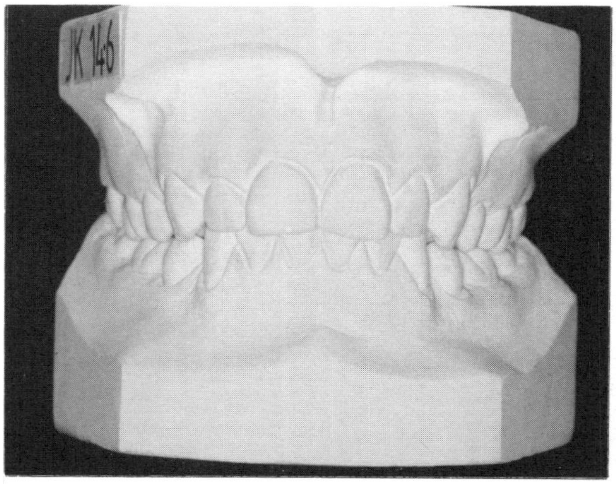

Appliance design

Palatal retractors were employed for the upper canines although this could have led to further rotation of these teeth as they were retracted and it might have been more appropriate to have used buccal retractors. The labial bow was included in the hope that the case could be completed with one appliance. There was no problem about anchorage (there was a half-unit excess space in the upper arch) and the reduced stationary anchorage effect which this component gives was not thought to be of significance. It should perhaps be pointed out that if the molars had not been fully intercuspated it would have been likely that any anchorage loss would have been accompanied by a worsening of the molar occlusion; if this had been the case molar tubes would have been included as a precaution.

The initial bite plane extended back 9 mm from the central incisor edges (i.e. overjet plus 3 mm) and was extended halfway up the palatal surfaces of these teeth. This was increased to full incisor height during the first 3 months of treatment. The acrylic distal to both upper canines was, of course, removed at the time of fitting.

COMMENTS ON TREATMENT

Treatment proceeded uneventfully. The lower incisors aligned in only 4 months and upper arch treatment was complete in a further 6 months. This included 2 months during which the labial bow was split to form a flexible labial retractor to align the upper central incisors. The two halves were then rejoined by soldering to form a rigid retainer. After the usual 6 months' regime of retention the appliance was discarded. There were no post-treatment changes apart from further extraction space closure. The models shown were taken 18 months out of retention. Space closure was finally complete by $16\frac{1}{2}$ years, by which time third molars were beginning to erupt in the lower arch.

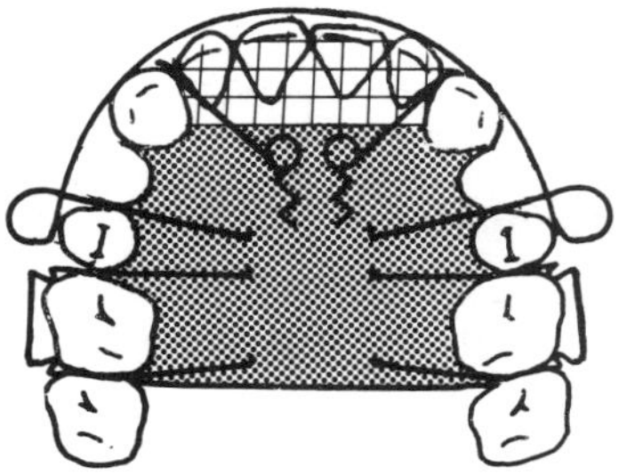

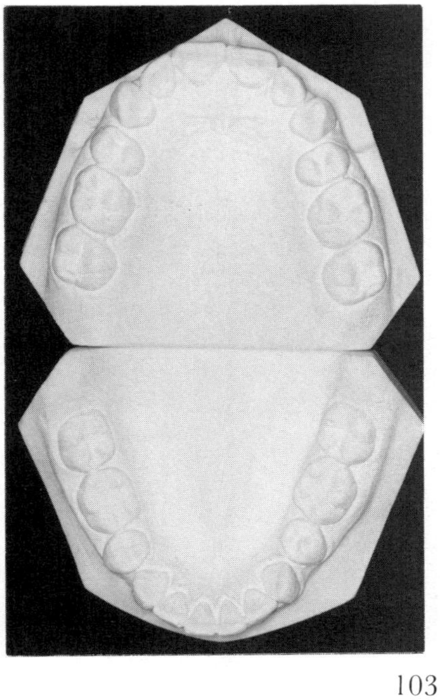

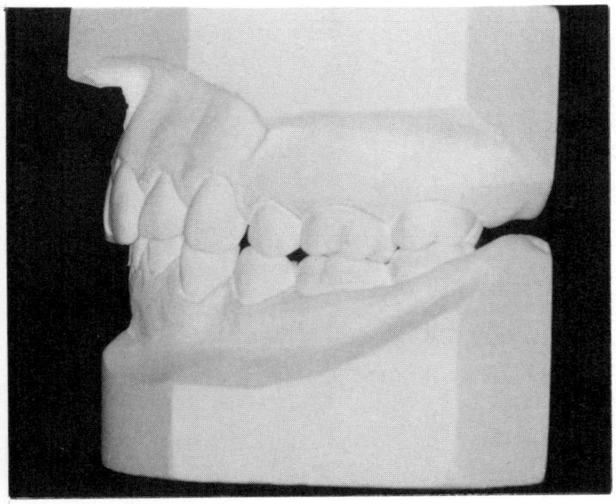

JA 14 years 3 months

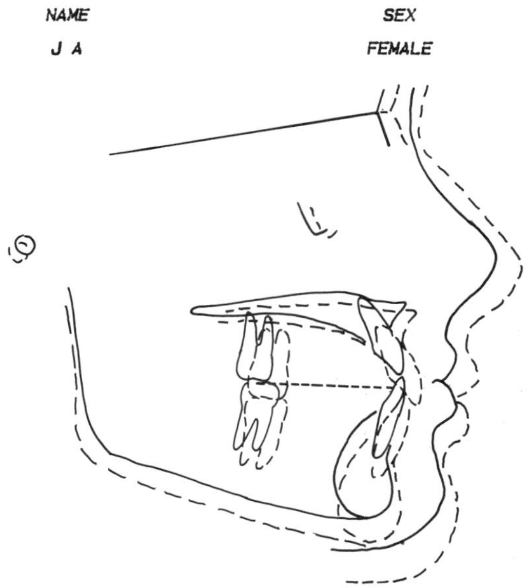

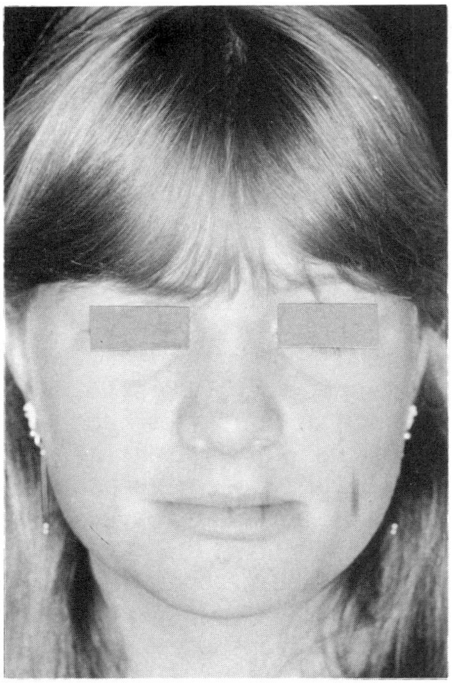

TREATMENT PLAN

Treatment aims

These were:

1 To correct the incisor relationship.
2 To maintain the space for the upper right second premolar if necessary.

Treatment means

Since the patient was unable to achieve an edge-to-edge incisor occlusion the prognosis was not particularly good. However, the overbite was not reduced and the lower incisors were slightly proclined and would therefore probably be stable after slight retroclination. It was felt that in the long term the patient would require upper and lower fixed appliance treatment and Class III traction and it would have been entirely reasonable to have delayed treatment until the premolars had erupted and this could be done. On the other hand present evidence suggests that the earlier a Class III incisor occlusion can be corrected the better is the ultimate prognosis for stability. Thus it was agreed to attempt correction with a short course of removable appliance therapy. This was possible because although lower incisor retroclination was required there was space in the lower arch to achieve this.

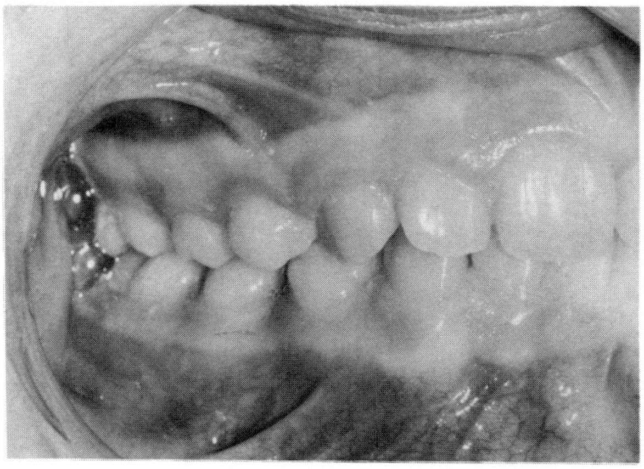

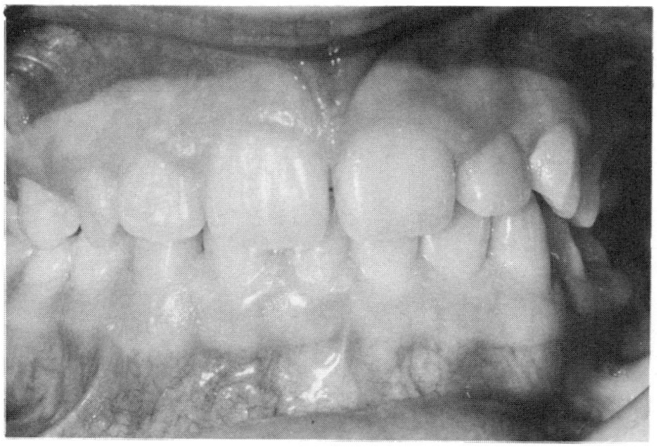

Appliance design

The simultaneous wearing of upper and lower appliances is seldom tolerated by the patient. Despite its surprising appearance an upper removable appliance carrying an inverted labial arch to engage the labial surfaces of the lower incisors is to be preferred and is usually extremely well tolerated. The appliance carries the usual Z-springs and posterior capping combination used for upper incisor proclination.

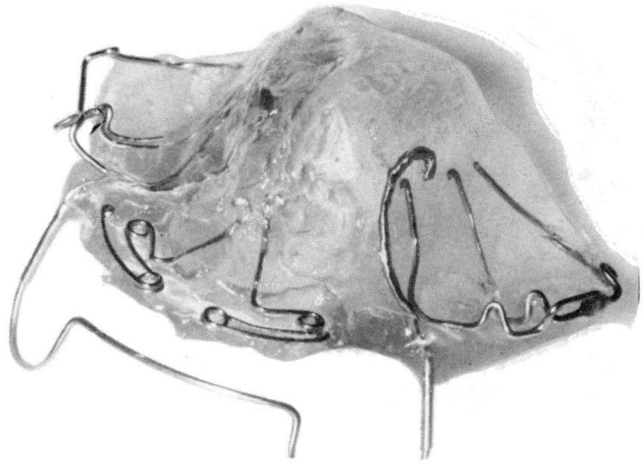

COMMENTS ON TREATMENT

The treatment proceeded far more quickly and achieved a much better result than had been expected. Treatment took just 2 months. There was no retention since the patient broke her appliance and failed to attend until 2 weeks later, by which time it was obvious that the occlusion was stable. The lateral incisors erupted into a Class I occlusion without intervention and no further treatment was required. The model shows the incisor relationship 4 months after correction. Photographs show the occlusion almost 4 years after treatment. It will be seen that the upper incisor centreline, although slightly improved, remains displaced to the right as a result of the premature loss of the upper right second deciduous molar. Fortunately this is not sufficient to affect the buccal occlusion.

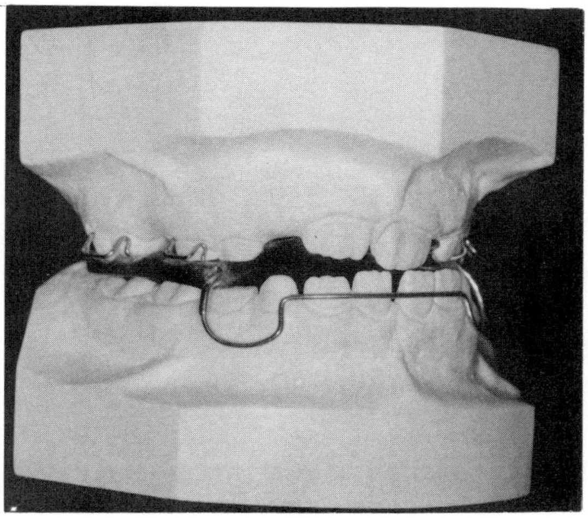

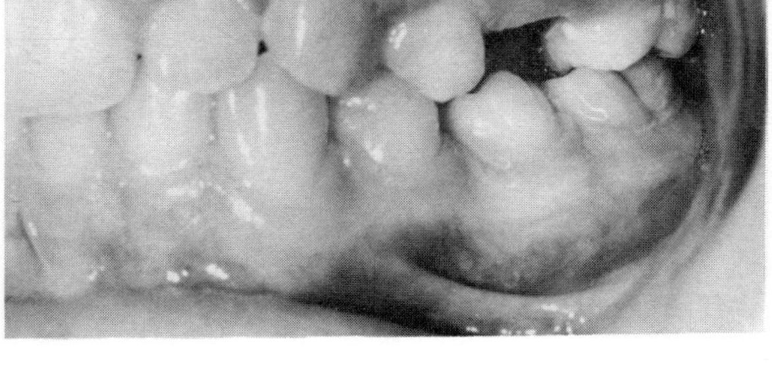

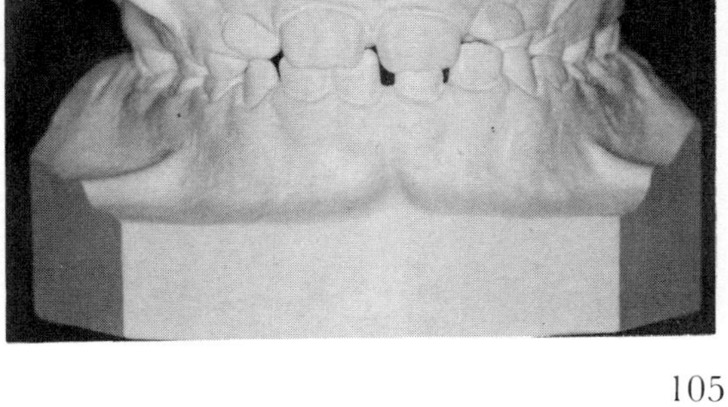

SN 14 years 3 months

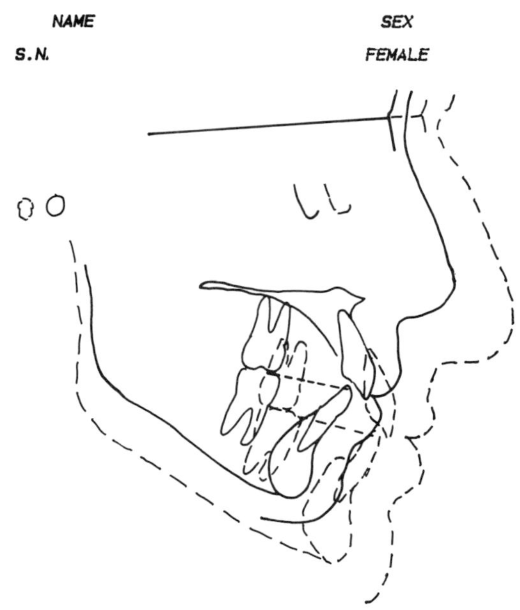

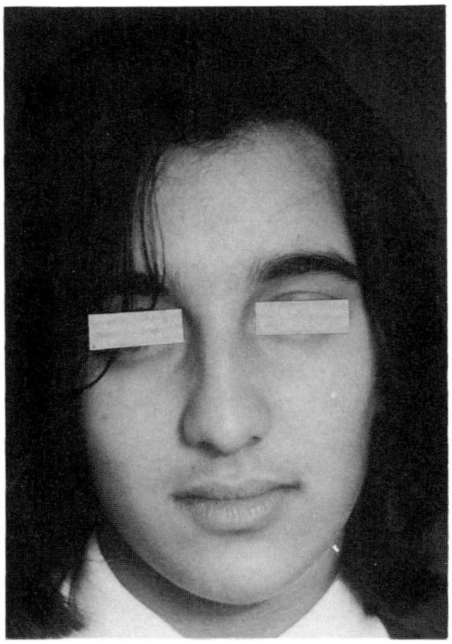

TREATMENT PLAN

Treatment aims

These were:

1 Improvement in oral hygiene.
2 Relief of crowding.
3 Alignment of the upper and lower labial segments.
4 Reduction of the overjet.

The bimaxillary proclination was to be accepted.

Treatment means

The crowding in the lower arch was judged sufficient to justify first premolar extractions but the marked distal inclination of the lower canines meant that little if any spontaneous improvement of the lower labial segment alignment could be expected. A lower fixed appliance was therefore considered obligatory and to a lesser extent, the rotation of the upper central incisors required fixed appliances to be employed in the upper arch also if a worthwhile improvement was to be obtained.

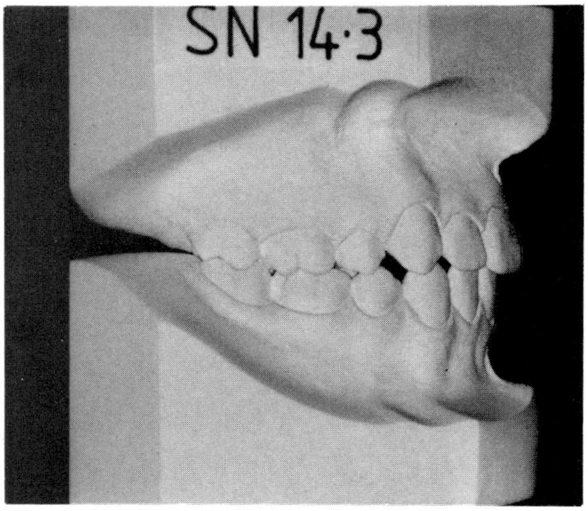

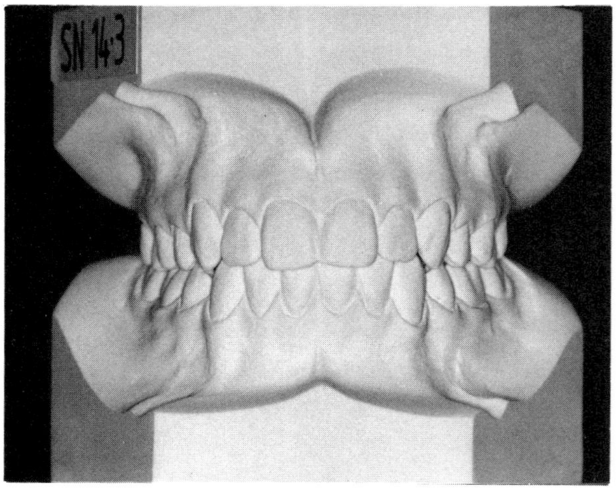

Appliance design

Straight-wire edgewise technique was employed. Headgear was used throughout treatment to maintain the Class I molar relationship in the face of considerable posterior stacking.

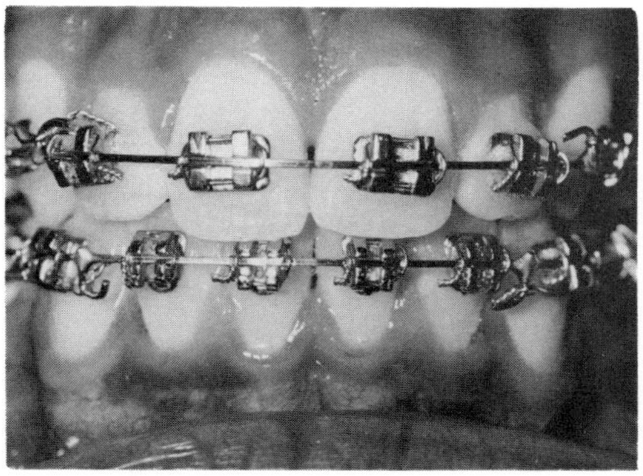

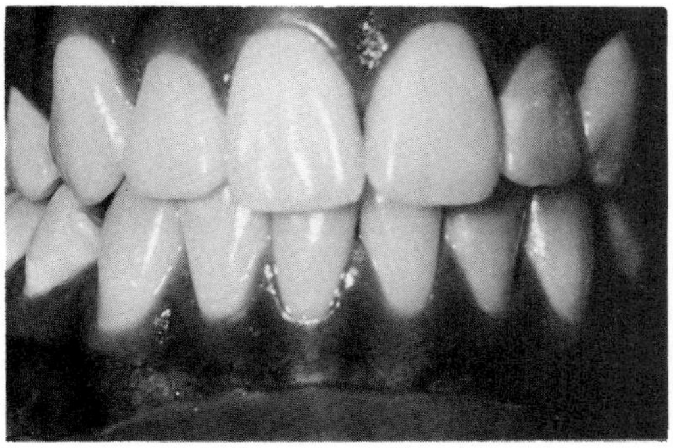

COMMENTS ON TREATMENT

The superimposed tracing shows remarkable forward growth of the mandible and lower face. Treatment was completed in 15 months and was followed by the usual retention period of 3 months full time and 3 months' nights only. The models show the occlusion 18 months out of retention.

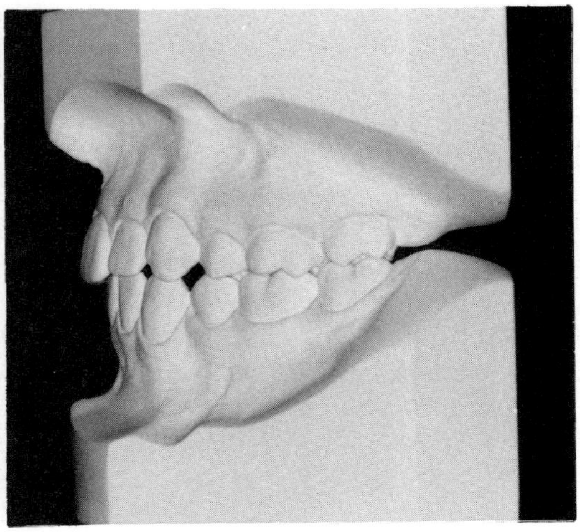

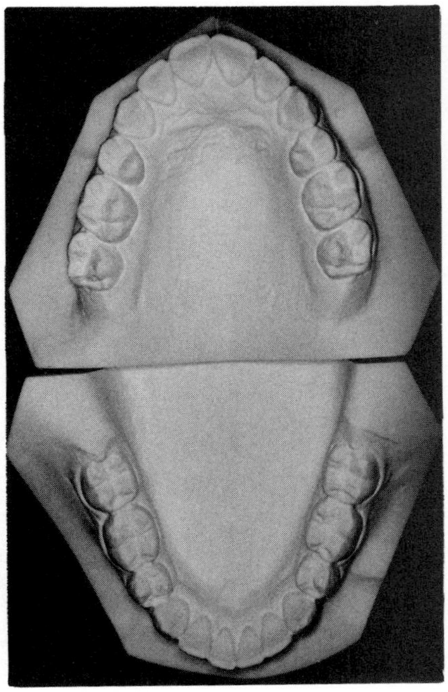

EH 16 years

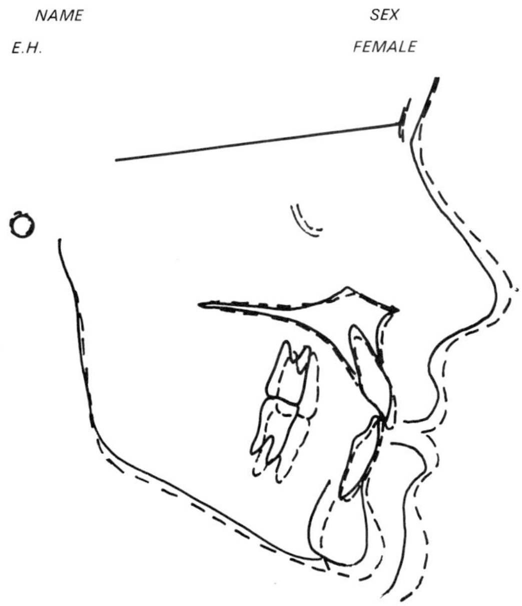

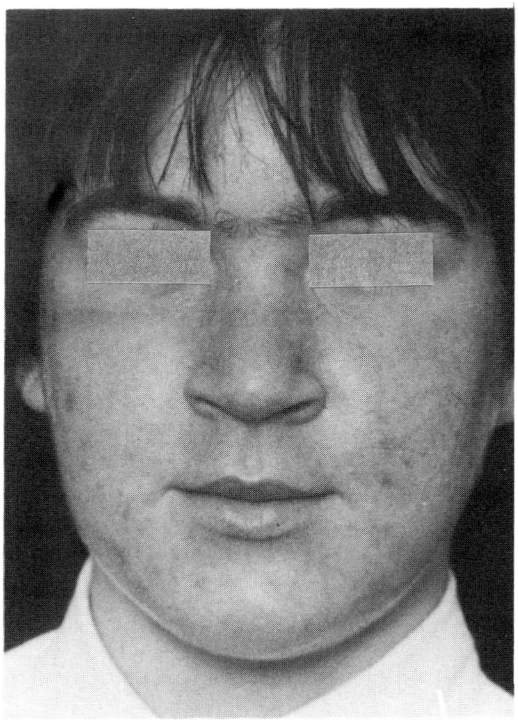

TREATMENT PLAN

Treatment aims

These were:

1 The elimination of the mandibular displacement through the correction of the instanding lateral incisors.
2 The relief of crowding.
3 The correction of the bilateral crossbite on the premolars.
4 Extraction space closure.

Treatment means

Although there was minimal crowding, it was felt that there was a need to retrocline the lower incisors in order to ensure sufficient overbite to maintain the upper lateral incisors in their corrected position. The lower third molars were present and there is a tendency for mild lower crowding to worsen in the growing patient. For these reasons extraction of premolars was thought to be justified. Nevertheless the excess space produced was sufficient to require active closure and so a lower fixed appliance was used. Second premolars were chosen since this would provide the most appropriate anchorage balance, giving less

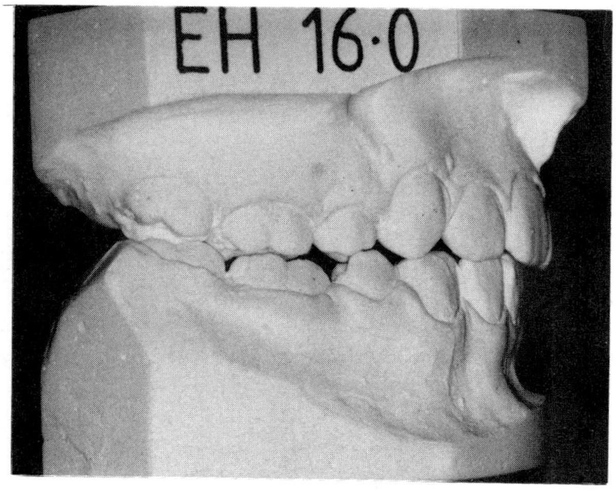

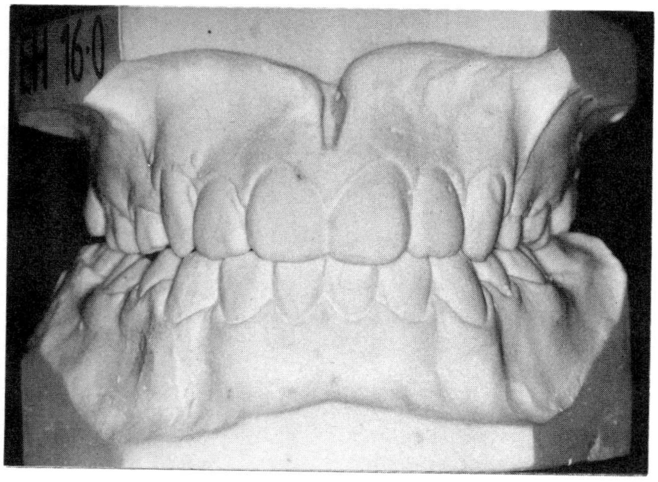

lower incisor retroclination during space closure than would occur with first premolar extractions. Also since fixed appliances were being employed there would be no risk of producing a poor first premolar – first molar contact.

In the upper arch the crowding required a full unit of space at the front of the mouth. This took precedence over the usual requirement of keeping extraction sites opposed and therefore upper first premolars were removed. In a Class III case headgear should be avoided for fear of worsening the skeletal discrepancy, hence in this case the need to preserve all the first premolar space was achieved by reinforcing the anchorage using intermaxillary Class III traction.

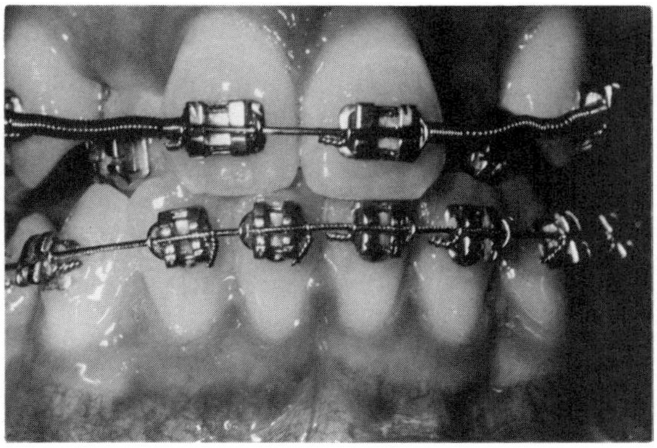

Appliance design

Straight-wire edgewise technique was employed. Pushcoils were used to recreate the space for the upper lateral incisors and reciprocally advance the central incisors over the bite. The use of fixed appliances avoided the common problem of overeruption and cuspal interference during space closure, which tends to occur where there are unmatched extractions.

COMMENTS ON TREATMENT

Treatment was completed in 21 months. The models show the case at this stage. The case was retained for a further year with removable retainers by which time growth was judged to have ceased. In view of the good overbite it is thought that the case is likely to remain stable.

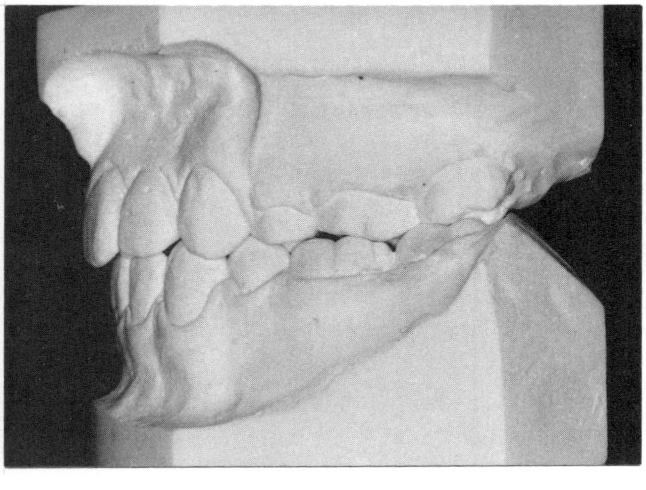

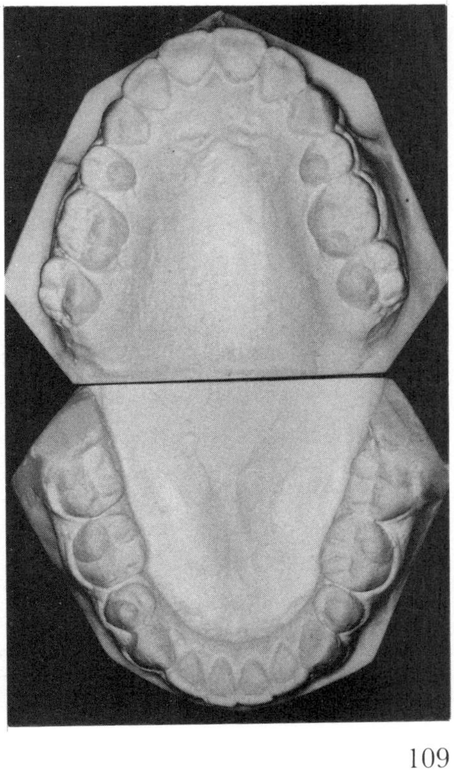

MB 14 years 1 month

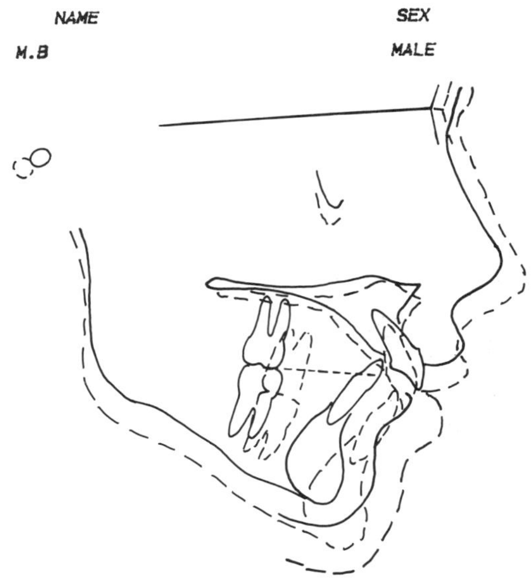

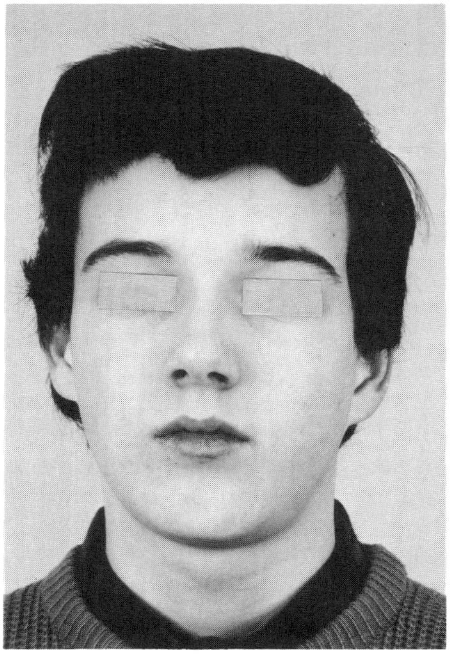

TREATMENT PLAN

Treatment aims

In the absence of crowding these were:

1 To correct the excessive overbite and overjet.
2 To correct the Class II molar relationship.

Treatment means

The severe skeletal class 2 dental base relationship, the absence of crowding and the patient's age suggested that a functional appliance might be used to good effect. This would have the further advantage that the appointments could be relatively infrequent and would overcome much of the problems of travel to the hospital. It was recognized that if this approach was unsuccessful, the combined problems of the severity of the skeletal pattern and the difficulty of travel would mean that a combined orthodontic–orthognathic approach was the only realistic alternative.

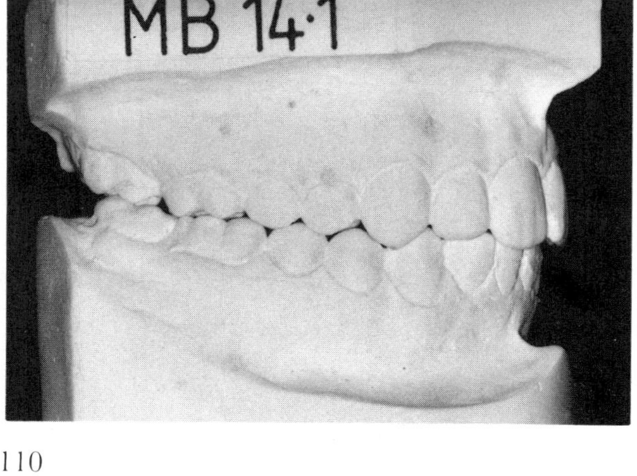

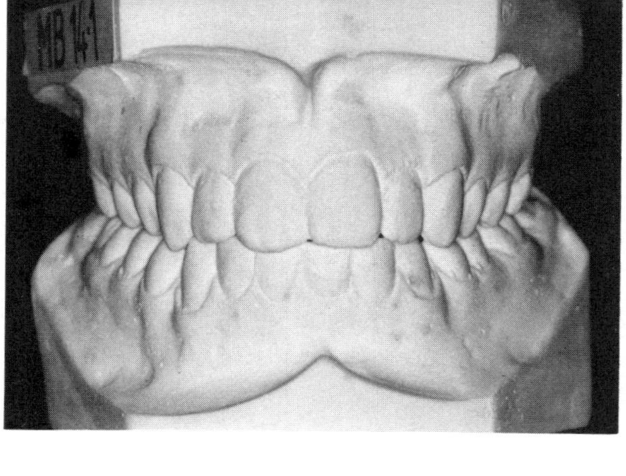

Appliance design

An activator of the Harvold pattern was employed.

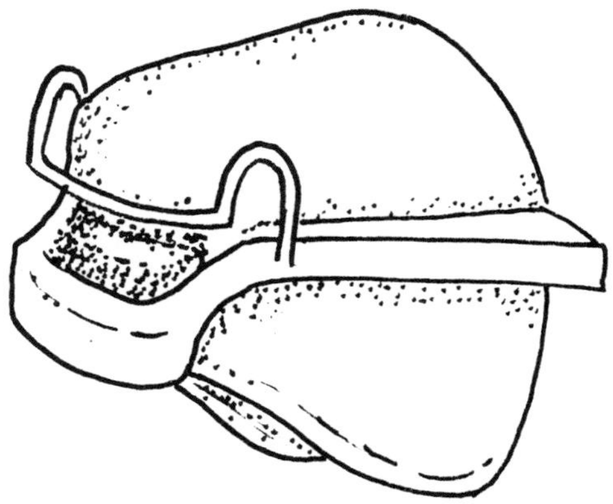

COMMENTS ON TREATMENT

Functional appliance treatment depends on the enthusiastic co-operation of the patient and the presence of favourable growth. In the event both these requirements were fulfilled and the patient had achieved an overcorrected Class III incisor relationship in 1 year – indeed, a short period with an upper removable appliance was needed to advance the instanding upper left incisor over the bite. The records show the case 18 months after the completion of treatment.

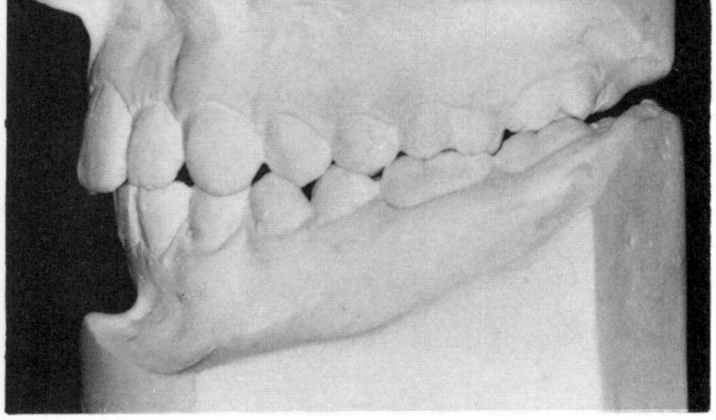

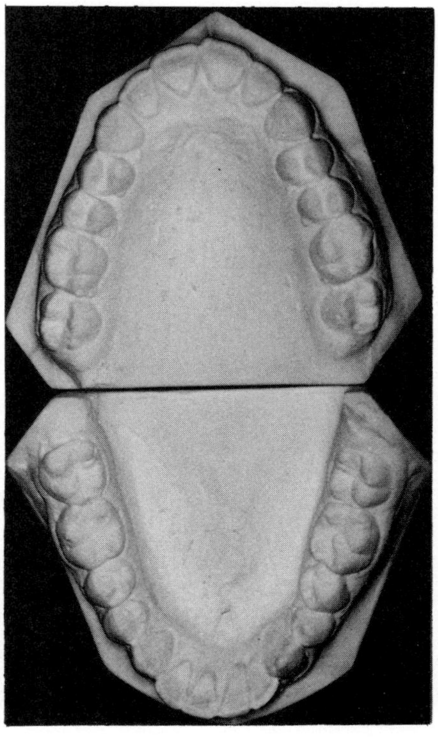

SR 16 years 6 months

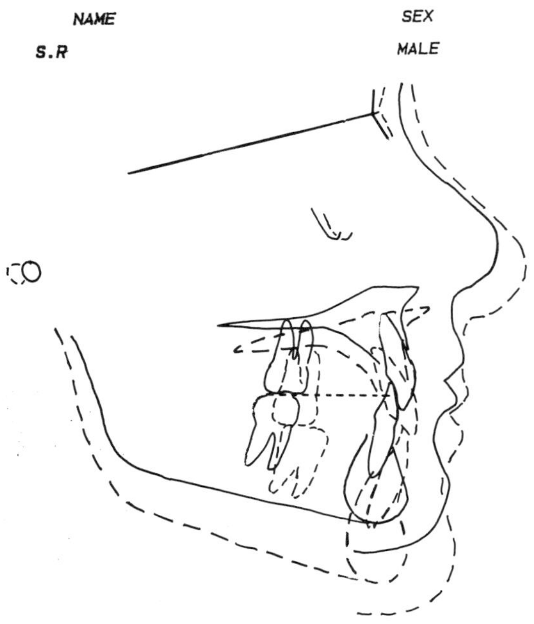

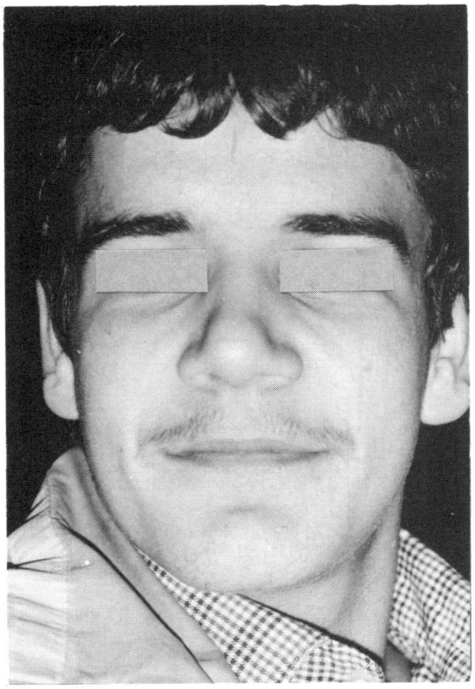

TREATMENT PLAN

Treatment aims

These were:

1 To relieve crowding.
2 To align the misplaced canines.
3 To correct the position of the upper lateral incisors and maybe correct the incisor relationship later if required.

Treatment means

The crowding was considered sufficient to warrant the extraction of first premolars. Space was quite critical on the right although on the left there might be some residual space unless subsequent spontaneous space closure was particularly favourable. It was thought wise to extract the upper deciduous canines with the three accessible first premolars to encourage the canines to align. (This would perhaps also encourage the lower centreline to correct as the unerupted premolars in the lower right quadrant attempted to erupt.) In view of the shortage of space on the right an upper space-maintainer was used.

It was felt that the canines had a good chance of erupting without surgical intervention and following their arrival an upper removable appliance could be used to align the lateral incisors if the Class II division 2 incisor relationship and the centreline displacement were acceptable at that time.

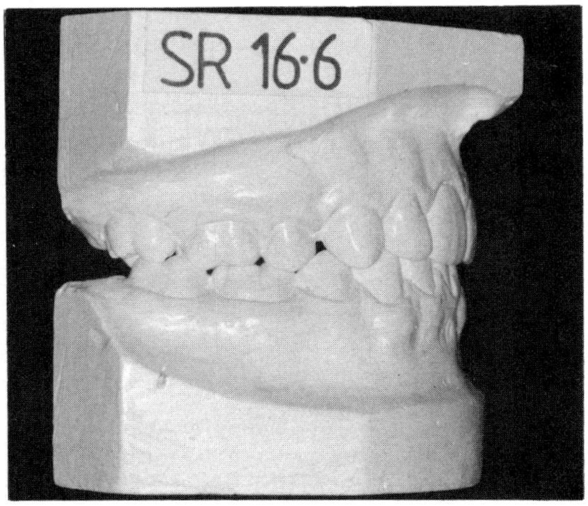

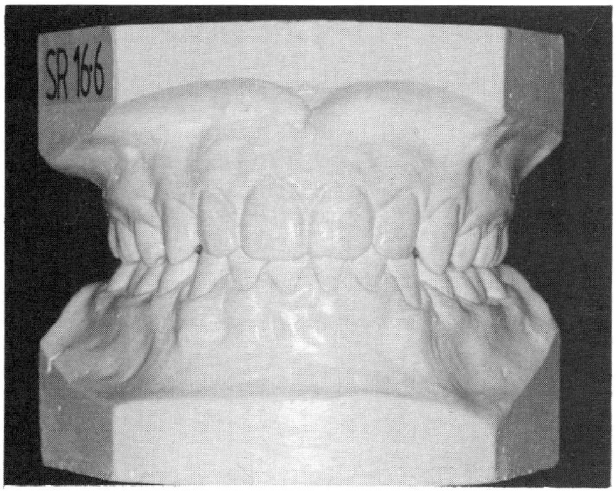

Appliance design

The removable appliance design was unremarkable. It was relieved widely in the premolar canine region to give minimum interference with canine eruption and in order to be as self-cleansing as possible. Once it was decided that fixed appliances were to be used, an anterior bite plane was added to assist in the overbite reduction prior to band placement (see below).

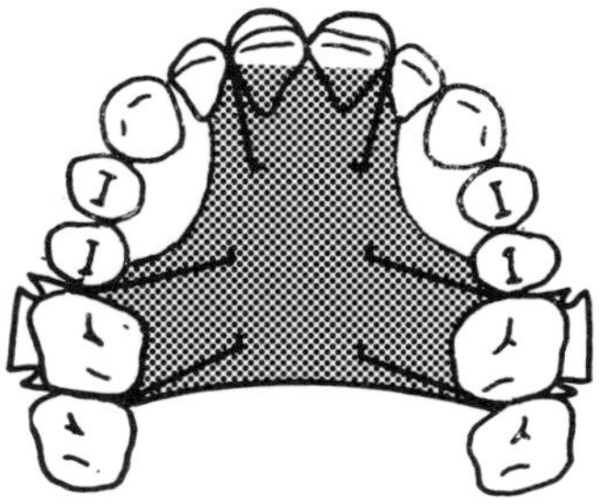

COMMENTS ON TREATMENT

Dental development proceeded very slowly. Six months after the extractions there was still no sign of the permanent canines but further intraoral radiographs showed their positions to be considerably improved. By this time the lower centreline was corrected and the lower right premolar had erupted and could be removed. By the age of 14 years 3 months the upper right canine finally appeared and was just buccal to its opponent. At this point the patient elected to undergo a course of fixed appliance treatment to obtain a rather better incisor relationship. A 1-year course of Begg treatment achieved a highly satisfactory result and was followed with 6 months' retention using a positioner.

The records are shown 1 year out of retention, shortly before all four third molars were surgically removed by lateral trepanation.

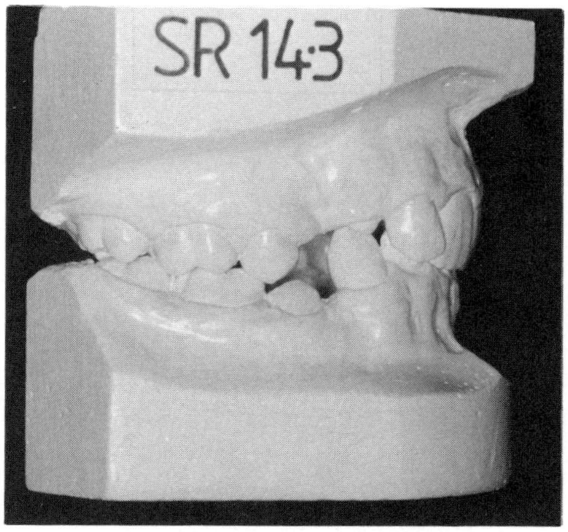

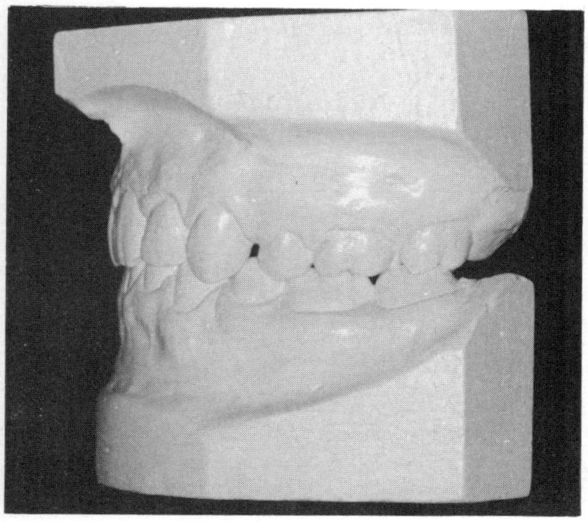

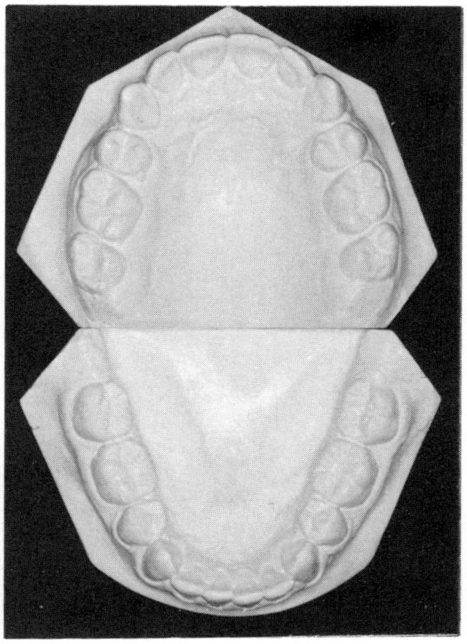

LM 14 years 7 months

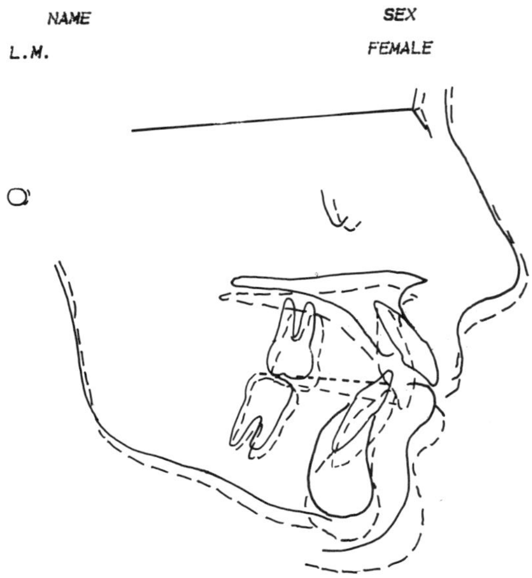

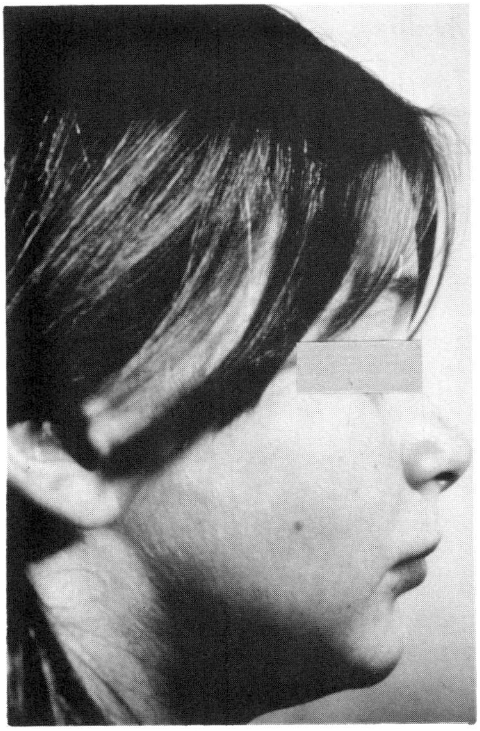

TREATMENT PLAN

It was felt that the alignment of the lower arch should be accepted.

Treatment aims

These were to reduce the overbite and overjet.

Treatment means

As the upper canines and labial segment were significantly proclined it was felt that an acceptable result could be obtained using maxillary removable appliances provided that the slight rotation of the upper right lateral was accepted. Since almost a full unit of space was required extraction of both upper first premolars was advised.

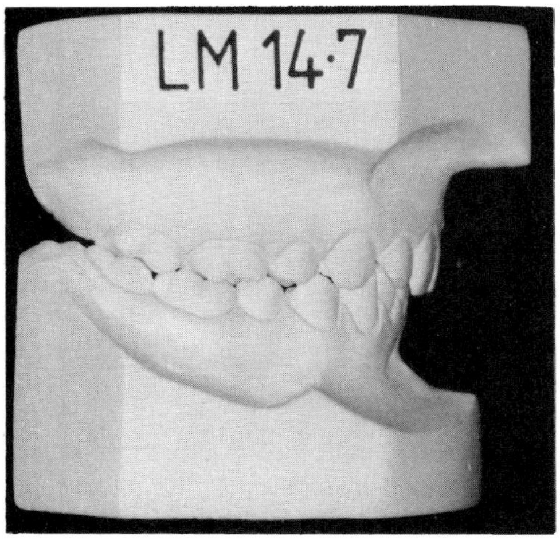

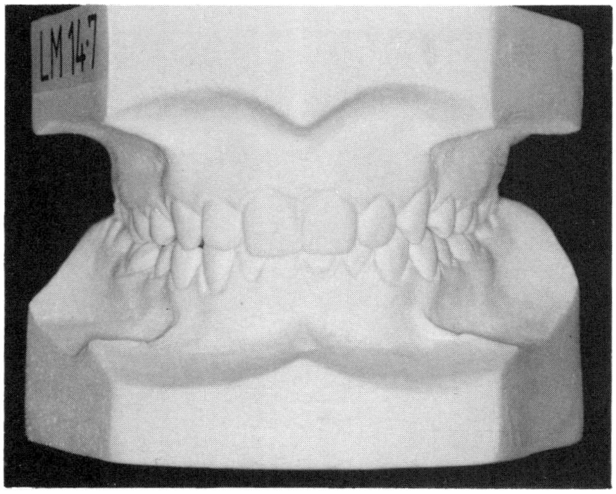

Appliance design

The appliances were designed to allow extraoral anchorage to be added if necessary, although it was recognized that some very slight mesial movement of the upper buccal segments would help to achieve a fully intercuspated Class II molar occlusion. The position of the canines allowed the preferred palatal retractor to be used in the first appliance. The second appliance utilized a Roberts retractor (0.5 mm high tensile wire supported by 0.5 mm i.d. tubing) as it was felt that the proclination of the upper incisors would cause a split labial bow to slide apically, with the risk of gingival trauma. As the flexibility of the Roberts retractor cannot be reduced to form a rigid retainer, at the end of incisor retraction a further appliance was required to do this. This was of identical design to the first appliance except for the omission of the palatal springs.

COMMENTS ON TREATMENT

Treatment proceeded uneventfully in two stages – canine retraction and overbite reduction, followed by reduction of the overjet. No significant anchorage was lost and headgear was not required. Tooth movement was completed in 12 months and was followed by the usual 6 month period of retention (3 months' full-time and 3 months' nights only wear). The models are shown 1 year out of retention. As with all cases of this kind, the slight retroclination of the upper labial segment causes the contact points to be more anterior than they would be in an ideal Class I occlusion. Hence if the canine is in contact with the lateral it too lies slightly mesial to a fully intercuspated Class I occlusion. The result is that if the molar occlusion is fully intercuspated, there is slight residual space distal to the canine (this is clearly preferable to having a disturbed molar occlusion). The more serious the skeletal discrepancy, the more retroclined the upper labial segment becomes, and the larger this residual space. In this case, if the lower incisors had not been so proclined, full overjet reduction could not have been obtained with removable appliances without producing unacceptable retroclination of the upper incisors with much greater residual space behind the canines.

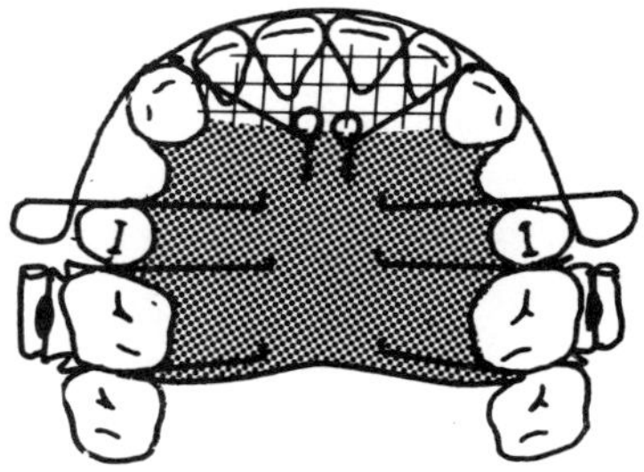

Appliance 1

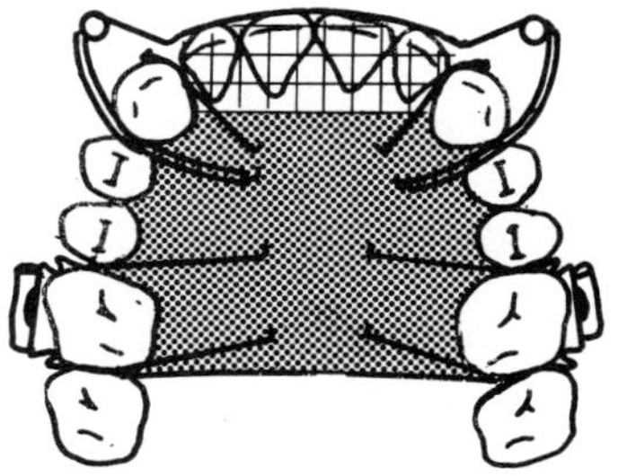

Appliance 2

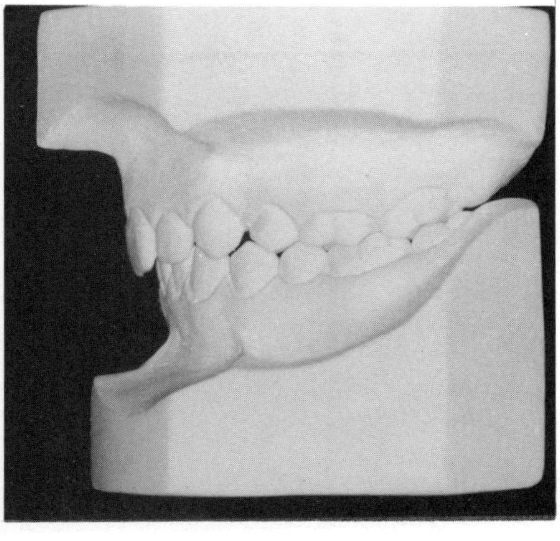

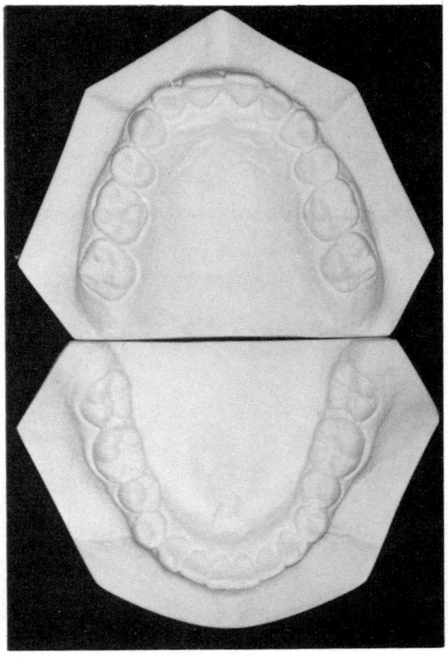

ML 13 years 10 months

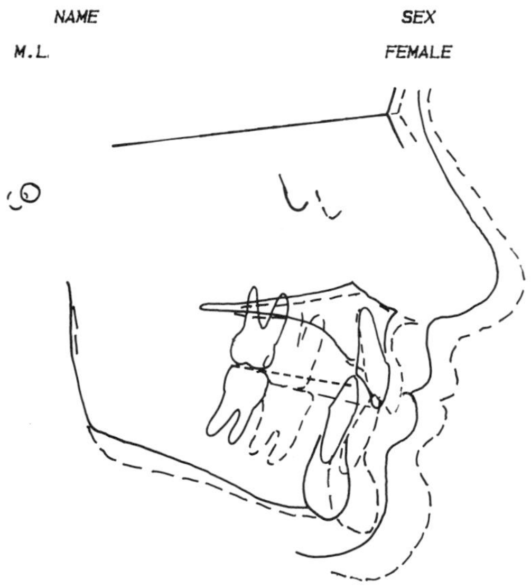

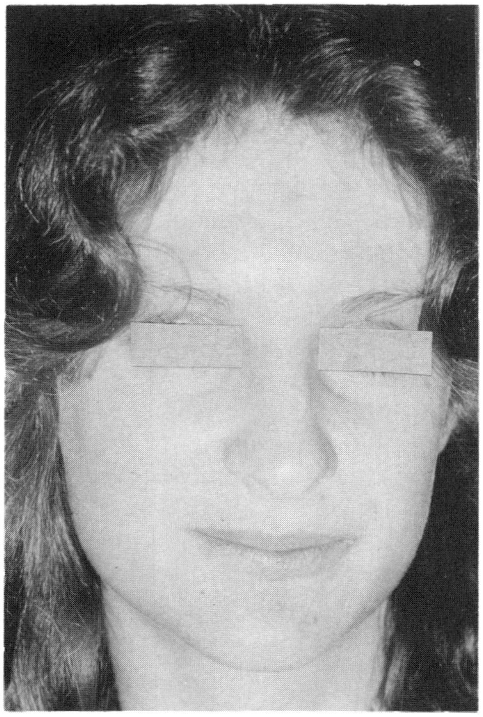

TREATMENT PLAN

Treatment aims

These were:

1 To relieve crowding.
2 To correct the incisor relationship and centreline.
3 To correct the molar occlusion.

Treatment means

The incisor occlusion, the unfavourable canine angulation in the lower arch, and the rotated upper lateral incisors all suggested that a fixed appliance would be required. Whilst the case might have been treated without premolar extractions it was considered that the form of the lower lip contraindicated further proclination of the lower incisors. First premolar extractions were decided upon, although in retrospect loss of the lower left second premolar and the first premolar in the remaining quadrants might have made treatment easier.

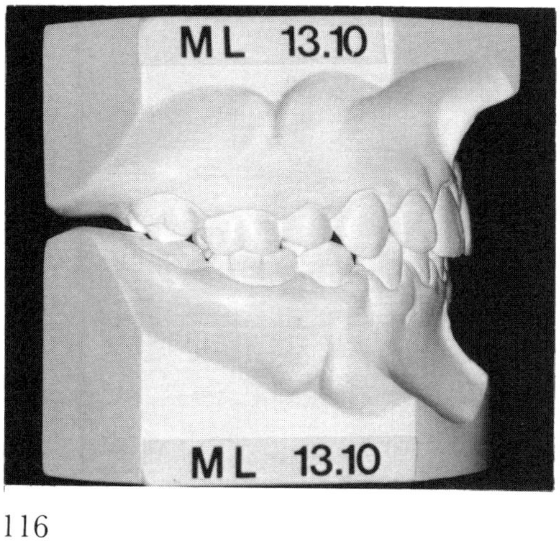

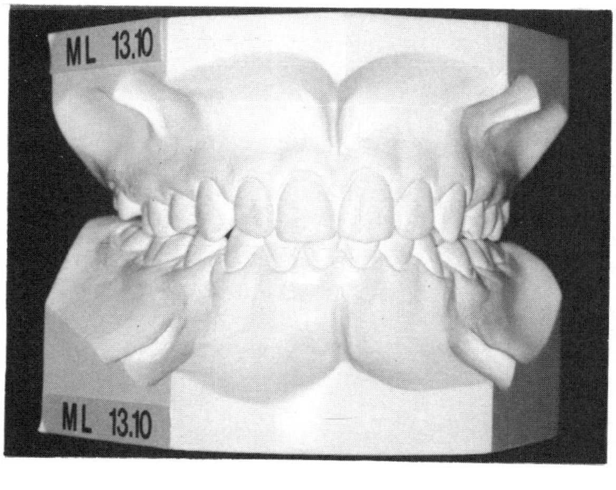

Appliance design

The case was treated using the Ricketts edgewise technique but could equally well have been treated with standard edgewise or Begg technique.

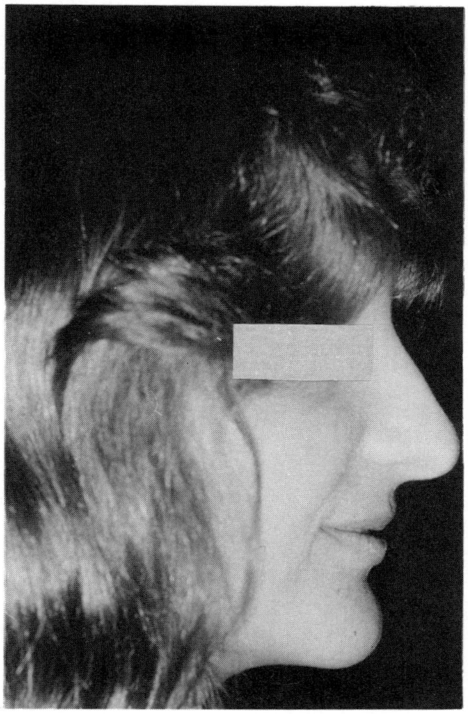

COMMENTS ON TREATMENT

Treatment took 1 year 10 months to complete. Extraoral anchorage was required to assist in molar correction. Overbite reduction was slow and post-treatment radiographs indicated that there was very little growth during this period, which probably accounts for both these difficulties. Centreline correction and space closure in the lower arch proved to be a further problem; as the space on the left was closed so the incisor centreline correction was lost. In the end although an acceptable incisor relationship was obtained, the molar occlusion remained a half-unit Class II. Facially the case still leaves a lot to be desired but such changes which have occurred can be seen to be the result of chin and nose growth. Records are shown 7 months after retainers were removed.

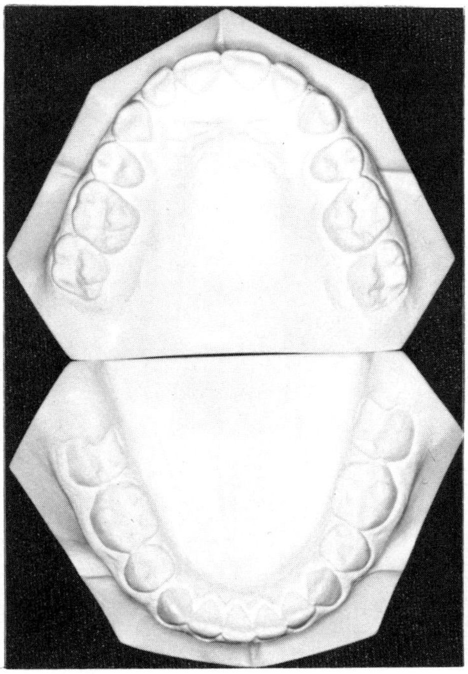

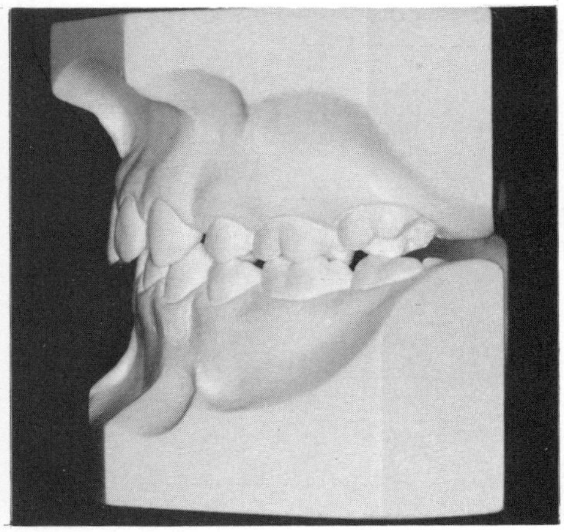

NO 15 years

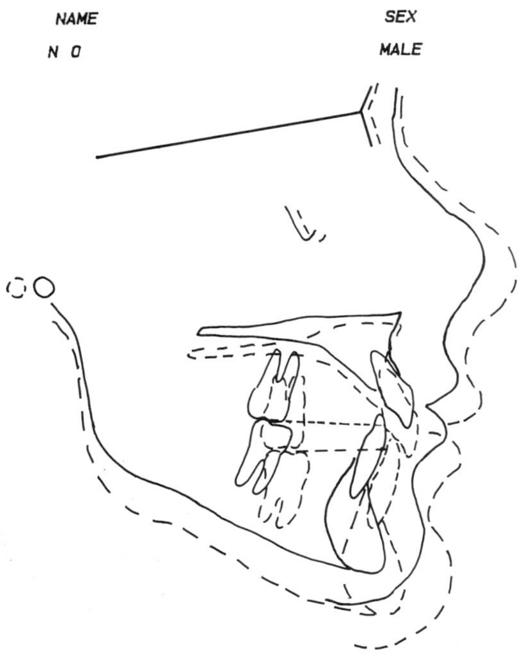

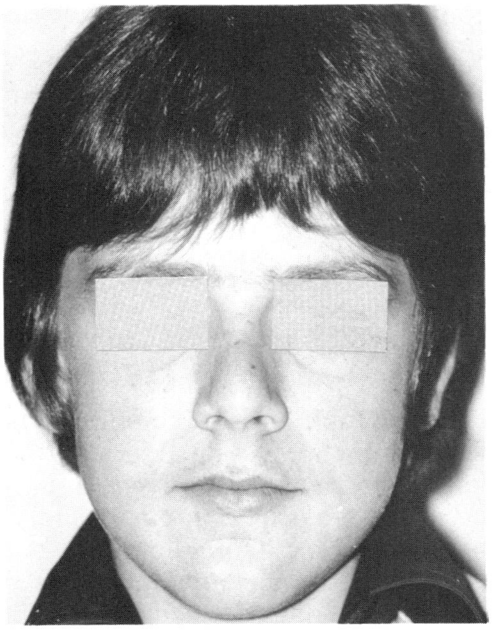

TREATMENT PLAN

Treatment aims

As the lower arch was considered to be acceptable and the position of the upper left central incisor did not give the appearance of excessive retroclination, the aims of treatment were alignment of the upper incisors, with reduction of the overjet where necessary.

Treatment means

The rotation of three of the upper incisors and the distal angulation of the right central incisor made a fixed appliance obligatory. It was felt that the overjet could be reduced by tipping movements and hence anchorage would not be a problem. Full overjet reduction was aimed at but it was thought that the upper left central incisor (overjet of 4.5 mm) was probably in a position of balance within the soft tissues and that there would therefore be some relapse at the end of treatment.

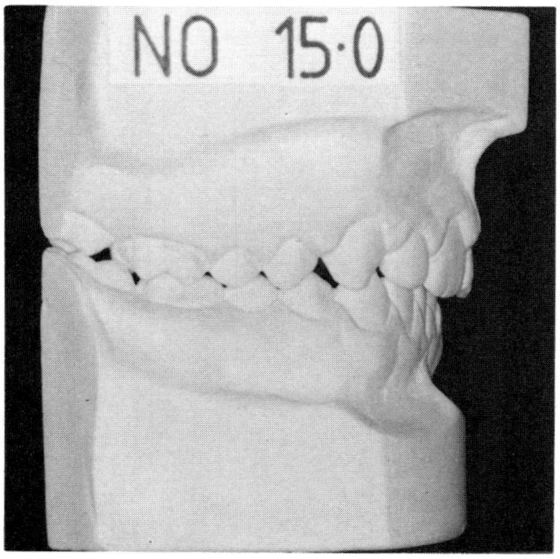

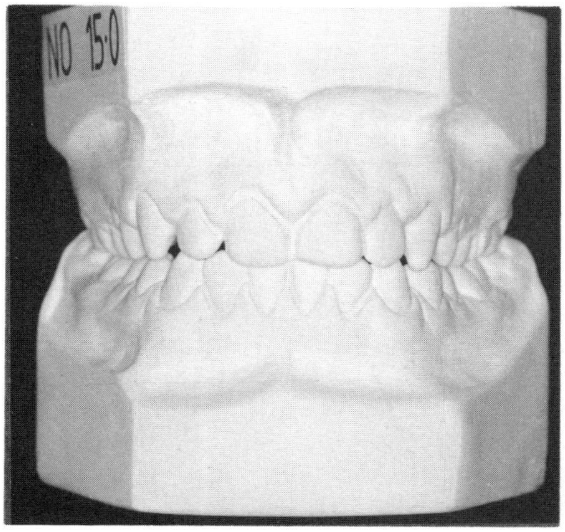

Appliance design

Begg brackets were used with light intramaxillary traction. It would have been rather simpler to have used edgewise brackets although the narrower Begg brackets allowed a multiloop arch to be employed, which achieved overcorrection of the rotations without an arch change.

COMMENTS ON TREATMENT

Overcorrection of the rotations was achieved within 5 months and the right central and left lateral were then pericised. Retention was carried out using an upper removable appliance designed to maintain these teeth in their overcorrected positions. The retainer was discarded after 6 months, following which there was a gradual increase of overjet to 5 mm.

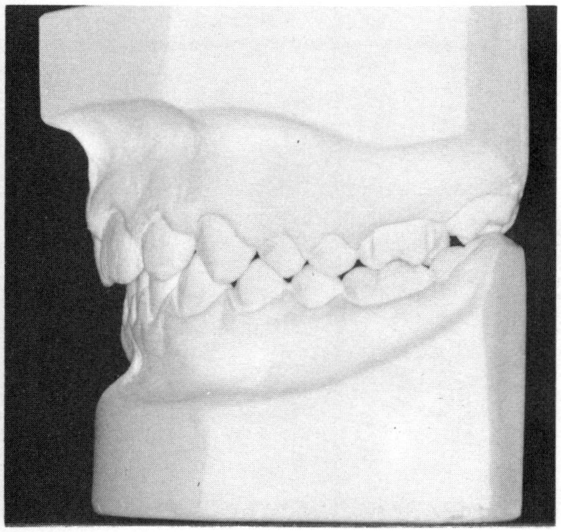

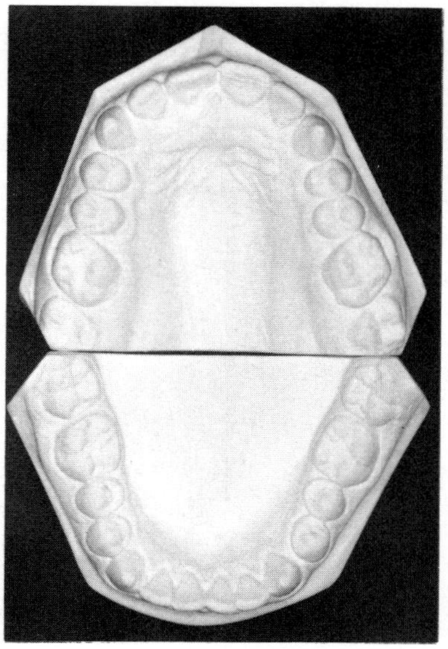

IR 16 years 3 months

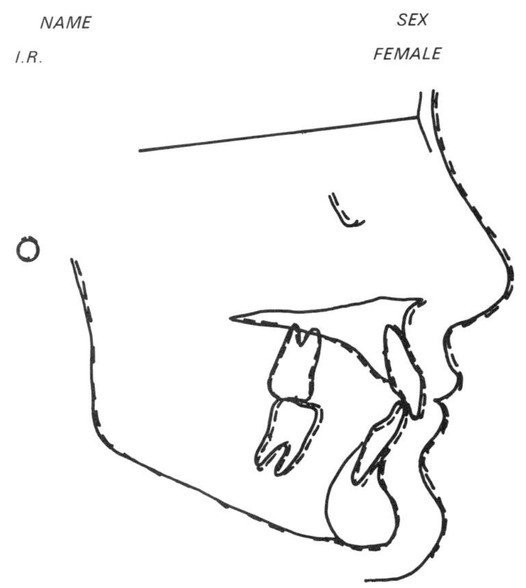

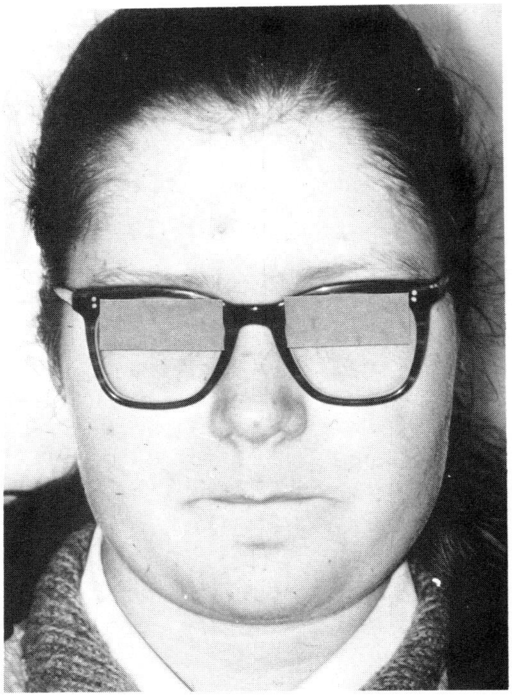

TREATMENT PLAN

Treatment aims

It was decided that the lower arch should be accepted. The treatment aim was therefore to align the upper lateral incisors.

Treatment means

The crowding in the upper arch was thought to be too slight to justify bilateral extraction but too great to be achieved merely by interdental reduction of the upper anterior teeth. Unilateral extraction of a premolar was briefly considered but it was thought that the resultant shift of centreline required to accommodate the contralateral tooth would be unacceptable. It was concluded that distal movement of the upper buccal segments using headgear would have the greatest chance of success and the least likelihood of causing harm. It was argued that 1 mm space could be achieved on the left before the buccal occlusion was disturbed and on the right 2 mm more could be found. Whilst this was not enough fully to resolve the problem, a 'super Class I' (mild Class III!) occlusion would be an acceptable situation to be aimed for. Should this prove to be unstable once appliances were withdrawn, a small amount of post-treatment interdental reduction of the upper anterior teeth might then be sufficient to permit good buccal occlusion without the reappearance of the anterior crowding.

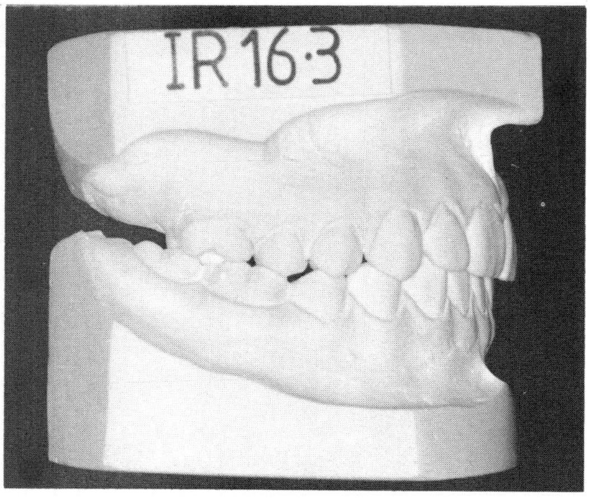

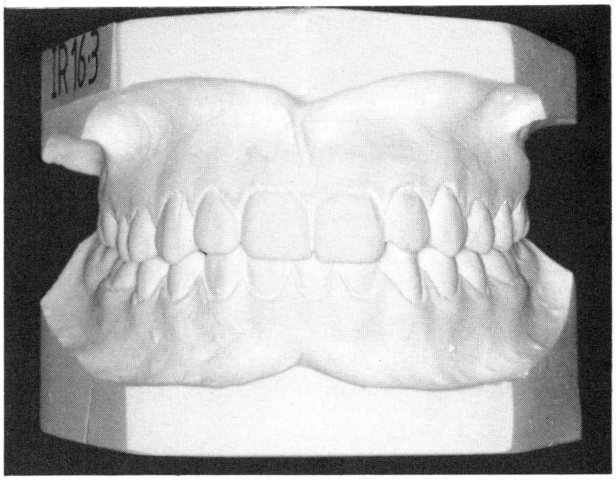

Appliance design

The first appliance was of the standard design used in retraction of upper buccal segments. A coffin spring is preferred by the authors to a midline expansion screw as it avoids relying on the patient to make the adjustment. It also allows differential anterior and posterior expansion should this be required. The head-gear tube is suspended on an auxiliary wire slung between the premolar and molar clasps in order to reduce the load on each. This has been found virtually to eliminate fracture of the clasps in use. There was no need for an anterior bite plane in this case and so the appliance was saddled to avoid any likelihood of a midline diastema occurring.

The second appliance maintained the extraoral anchorage while the lateral incisors were aligned. There was no need to retract the canines as these had followed the other buccal teeth distally, hence only stops were required mesial to these teeth. In the final stages of alignment these were removed to permit the lateral incisors to be fully accommodated.

COMMENTS ON TREATMENT

The buccal segments moved rapidly and adequate space had been produced within 5 months. Active treatment was completed in 10 months and was followed by the usual 6-month period of retention using the same appliance. During this time the lateral incisors were pericised and the upper second molars extracted. (The appropriateness of both these procedures is debatable but they were seen as a 'belt and braces' approach to reduce the degree and speed of any post-treatment relapse.)

Finally, selective grinding was carried out to achieve the best possible buccal occlusion. Much to everyone's surprise there was no detectable change following the discarding of appliances. Models are shown 1 year out of retention.

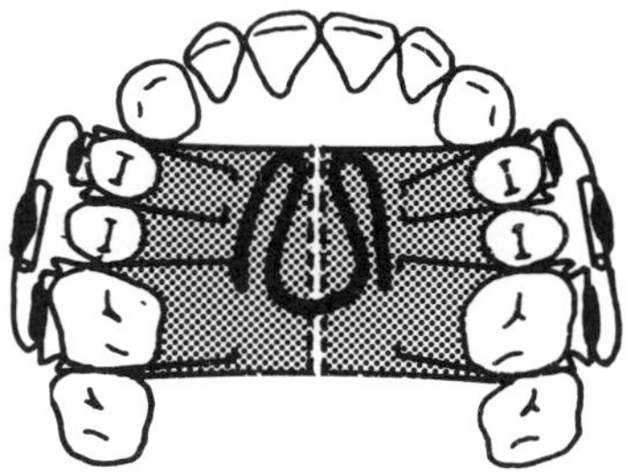

Appliance 1

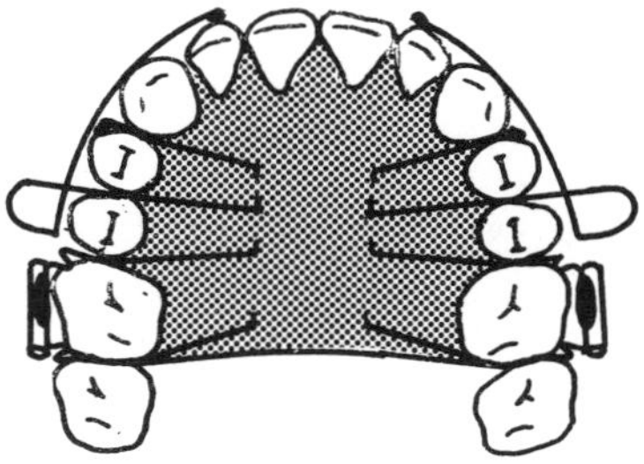

Appliance 2

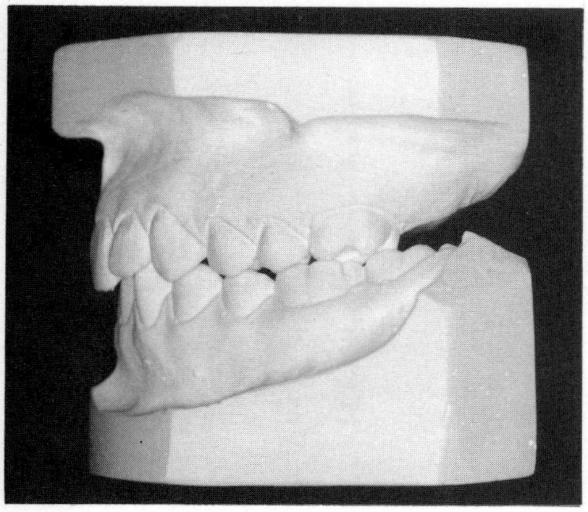

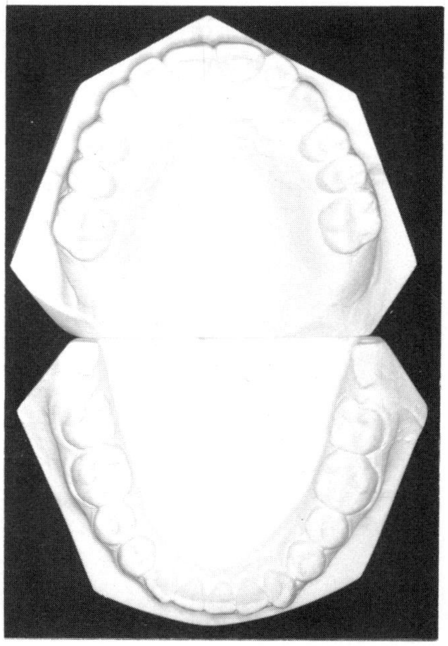

ATh 13 years 5 months

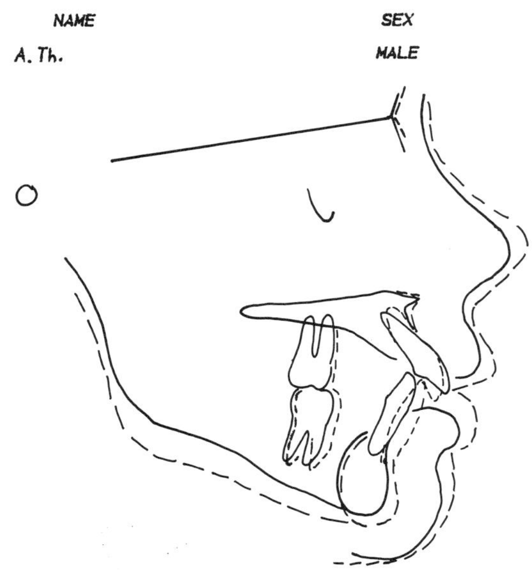

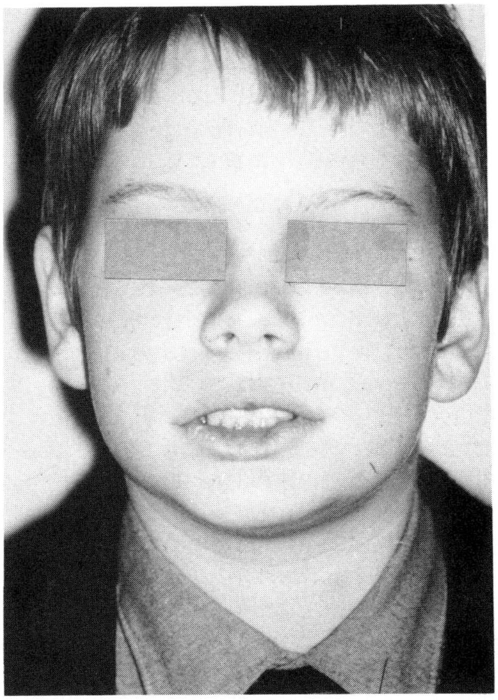

TREATMENT PLAN

Treatment aims

It was felt that nothing could be done without a marked improvement in the oral hygiene. Treatment aims were therefore:

1 To improve the oral hygiene and arrest active caries.
2 To discourage the thumb habit.
3 To reduce the overbite and overjet.

Treatment means

Dietary control and fluoride application made a significant improvement to the level of caries activity and initially the oral hygiene showed a marked improvement. It was felt that treatment should be kept simple. The lower arch was accepted and an upper removable appliance fitted to discourage the digit habit. Once this had been achieved, canine retraction and overjet reduction were undertaken using the available space. As there was only just sufficient space to make the canines Class I there was every indication for extraoral anchorage to be used.

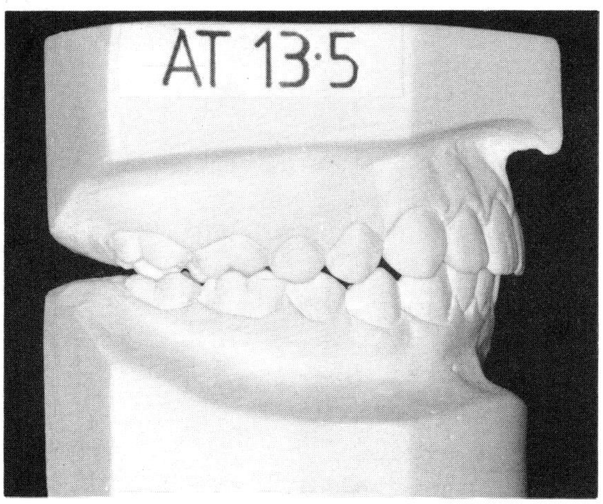

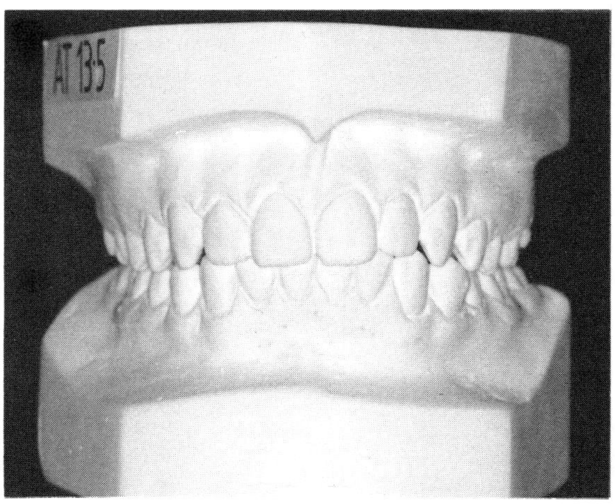

Appliance design

A typical appliance was used incorporating palatal springs (0.5 mm) for canine retraction and a labial bow which could later be divided to form two flexible incisor retraction arms.It should be noted that where such a bow has closed U-loops it should be made out of 0.8 mm wire to offset the increase in flexibility which this design provides. The molar clasps had soldered tubes attached to receive headgear should this prove to be necessary.

The anterior bite plane was half incisor height initially and was increased with cold-curing acrylic to full upper incisor height during the first 3 months of treatment.

COMMENTS ON TREATMENT

As has already been mentioned, the case warranted extraoral support of the anchorage. Initially, because of an extreme reluctance on the part of the patient to accept headgear, treatment begin without this. Canine retraction took 3 months, during which time overbite reduction had been completed. Only 3 months' incisor retraction was possible before all available space had been used up. By this time the overjet was 6 mm and the buccal occlusion almost a half-unit Class II. At this point the patient was convinced of the need to wear headgear and this was fitted.

Final overjet reduction was rapidly achieved without further activation of the bow; in other words, mandibular growth and distal movement of the entire upper arch were responsible. The appliance was discarded after 6 months' retention, during which period the two arms of the bow were rejoined by soldering. The models shown were taken 1 month after the appliance was discarded.

The tracing shows that the upper incisors underwent classical tipping around the middle third of their roots and the patient ended up with an ideal Class 1 incisor relationship. This was possible because the skeletal relationship was Class 1 and such sagittal discrepancy as existed was offset by the slight proclination of the lower incisors.

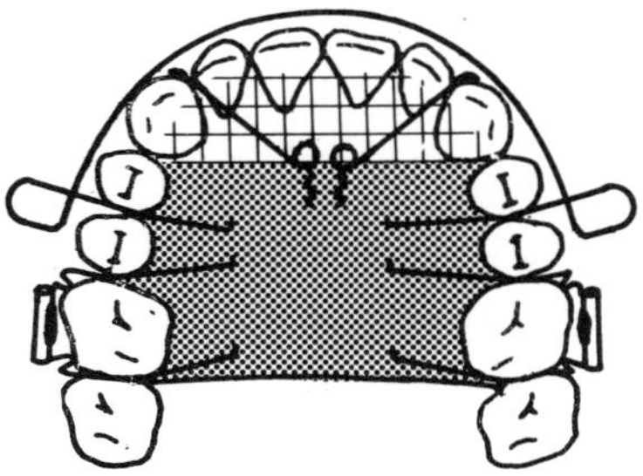

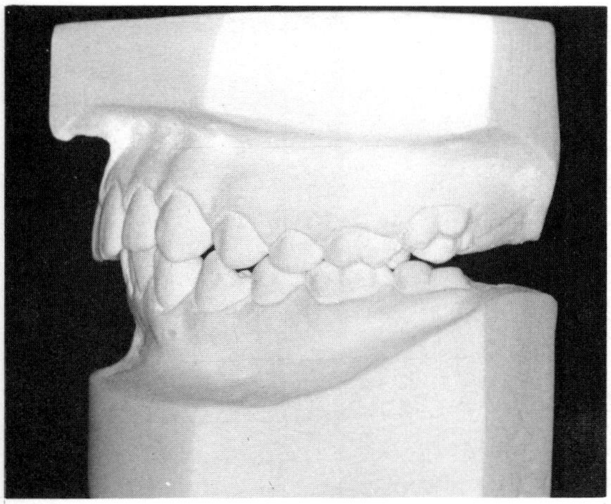

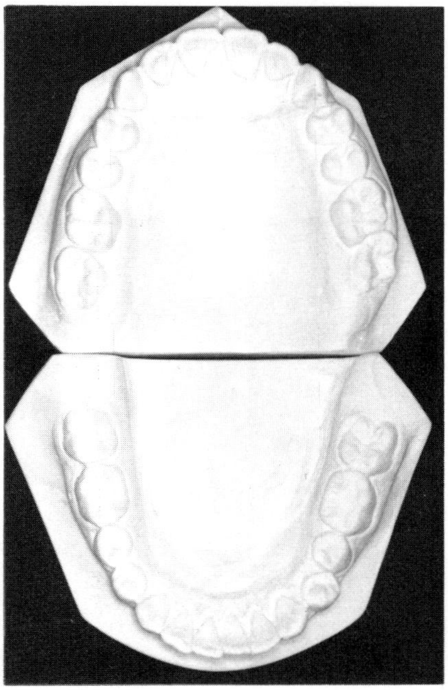

LJ 15 years 1 month

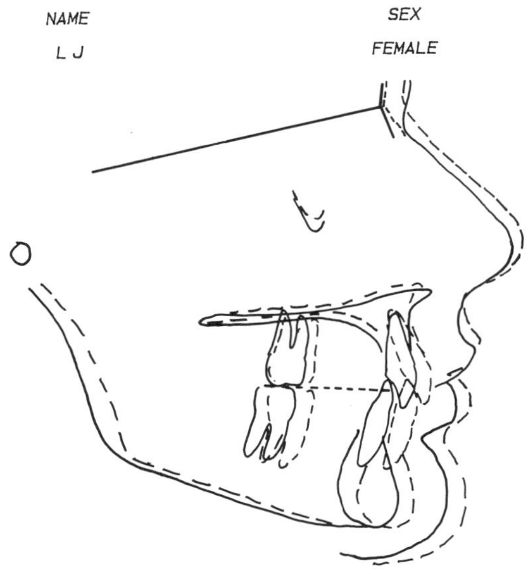

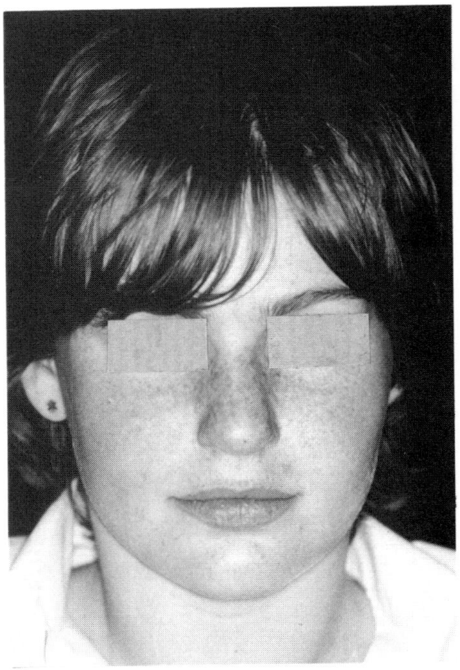

TREATMENT PLAN

Treatment aims

These were:

1 Reduction of the overbite.
2 Alignment of the upper incisors.
3 Establishment of a more satisfactory inter-incisor relationship.

Treatment means

Treatment of this kind of case is not easy. In a non-growing adult it would be on the border-line of what can be achieved by orthodontic means alone. However in the prepubertal child, given favourable growth, the underlying problem of the sagittal jaw relationship can sometimes be improved dramatically using a myofunctional appliance. It should be emphasized that this is not always successful and so the operator should have at his disposal the clinical skills to enable him to go over to fixed appliance techniques and treat the case conventionally (in this instance on a non-extraction basis with headgear support) if necessary.

Appliance design

Because of the need to adopt a forward postured bite to obtain sagittal jaw correction the

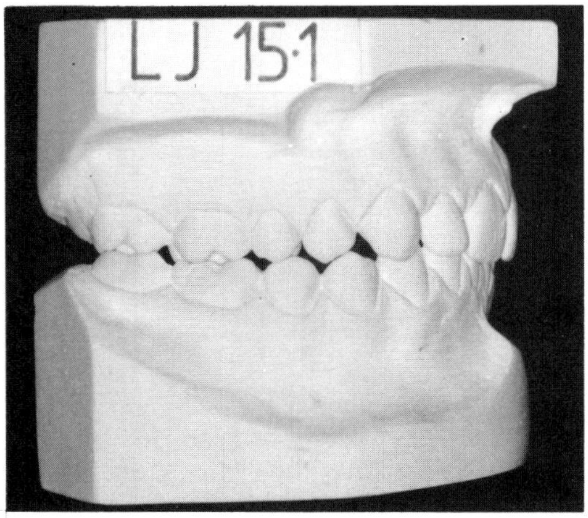

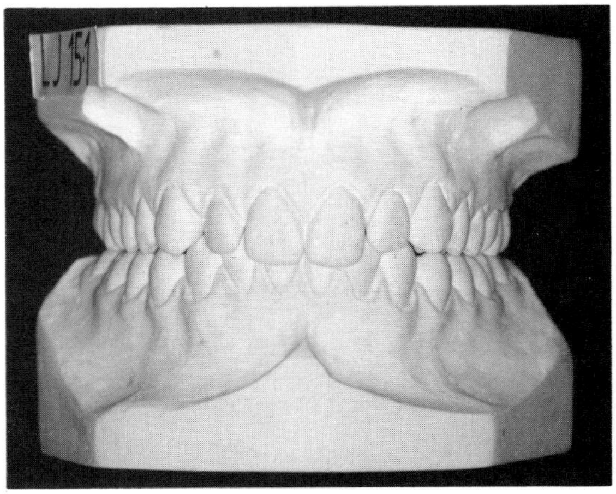

upper incisors must first be proclined. In other words the patient must be converted into a Class II division 1 case. Most people prefer to do this initially with a removable upper appliance worn full time as this helps overbite reduction. However in LJ's case there were already signs that she was entering her growth spurt and so the option of incorporating proclination springs in the activator was adopted. Flapper springs were placed in the acrylic behind all four upper incisors and because of the displacing effect which these have cribs were incorporated on first molars. Lower incisor capping covered the incisal half of the lower incisors both to prevent their eruption and to limit the tendency for these teeth to procline reciprocally during myofunctional treatment.

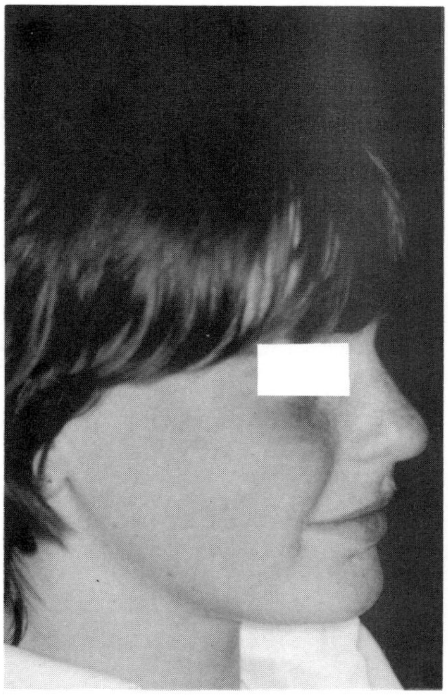

COMMENTS ON TREATMENT

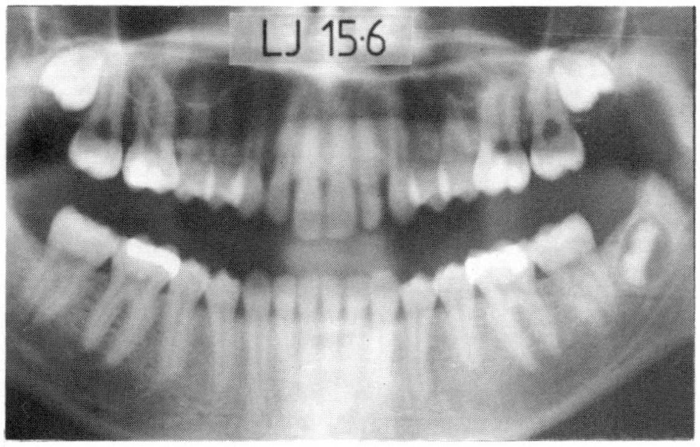

The patient tolerated the appliance well and proclination went hand in hand with sagittal correction. This was completed in fifteen months and was followed by a short period in which an upper removable appliance was used to improve the alignment of the upper lateral incisors. (Ideally an upper fixed appliance with headgear support should have been used but the patient was not prepared for this to be carried out and was keen for treatment to be concluded as soon as possible.) Treatment was completed in 20 months and the models shown were taken at the end of active treatment.

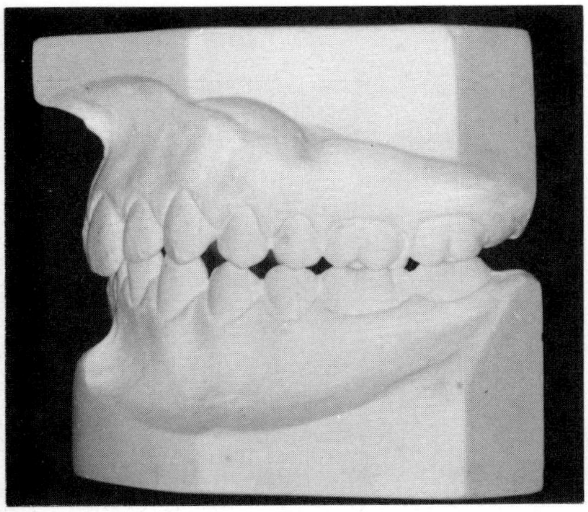

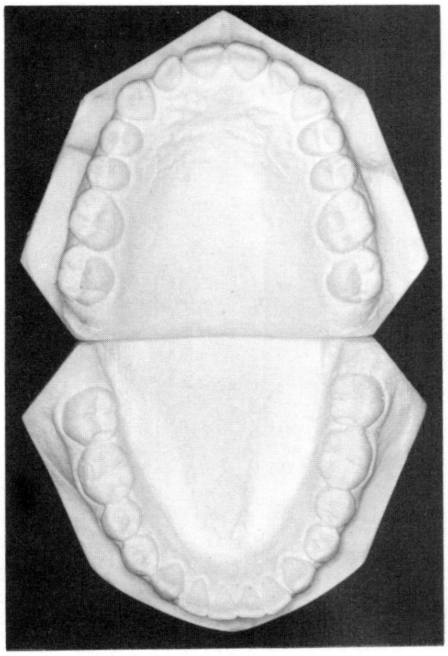

JS 14 years

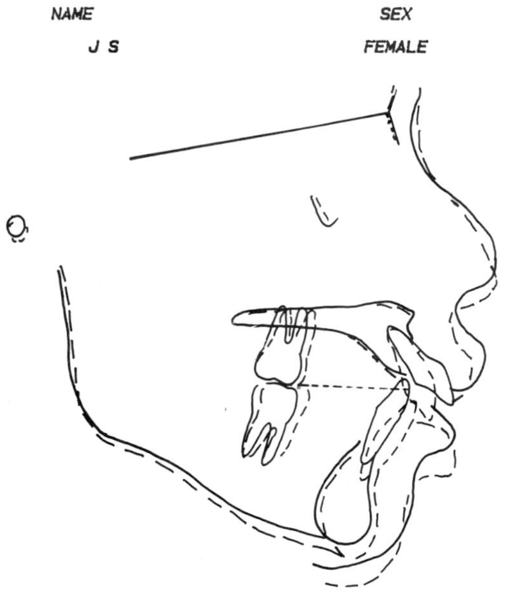

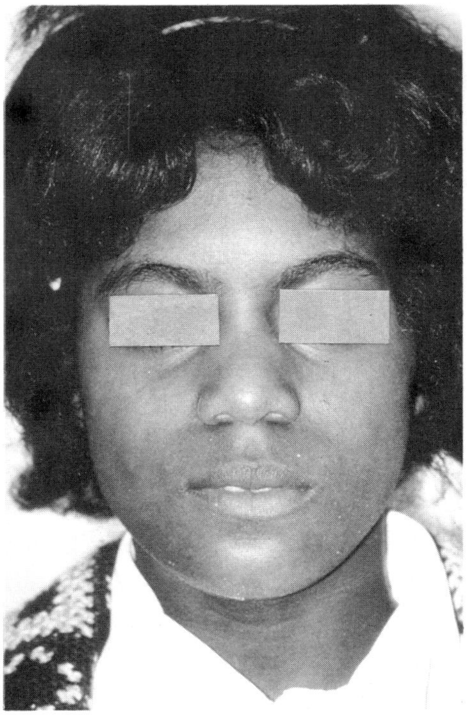

TREATMENT PLAN

Treatment aims

These were:

1 To improve the oral hygiene.
2 To accept the lower arch.
3 To reduce the excessive overbite and overjet.

Treatment means

The patient was still immature for her age and as the dental bases were long and there was no sign of posterior crowding it was felt that there was a good chance that the case could be treated satisfactorily with removable appliances by a combination of distal movement of the buccal segments followed by retroclination of the upper incisors. Success would depend upon good co-operation and favourable growth but it appeared that nothing would be lost by attempting treatment on this basis. If growth was unfavourable incisor retraction could be undertaken with fixed appliances, provided that the oral hygiene had improved in the meanwhile.

Appliance design

The first appliance was that typically used for distalization of buccal segments. The appliance is retained by clasps on the first molars and premolars, to which the support wire tube for the intraoral part of the face bow is attached. This arrangement reduces the like-

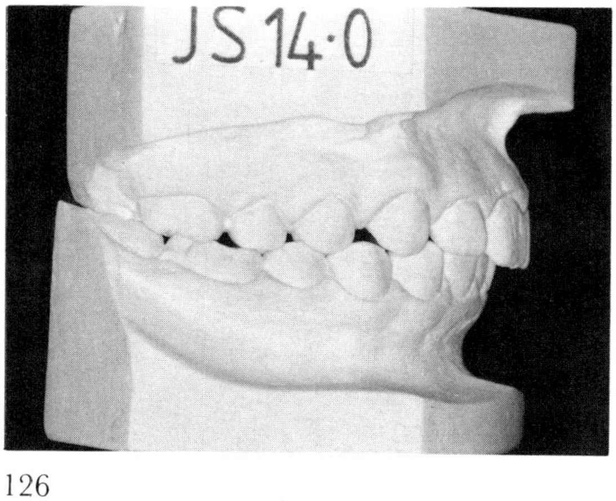

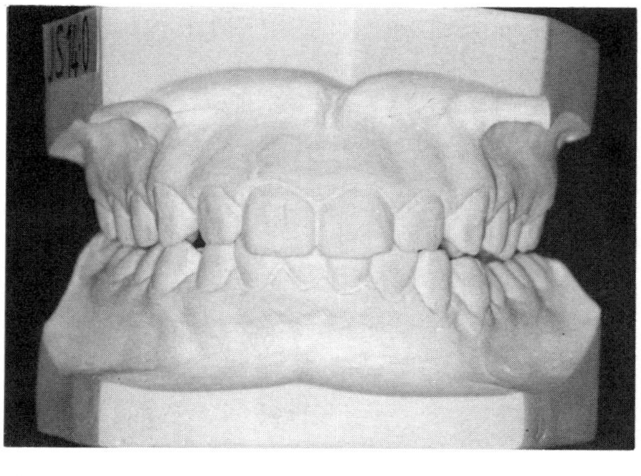

lihood of fracture of the clasps in use, presumably by reducing the level of mechanical stress on any one wire.

A coffin spring was used to maintain the correct interarch occlusion; this is preferred to an expansion screw because it does not require the patient to remember to turn it and the arch may be differentially expanded anteriorly and posteriorly.

Because of the excessive overbite an anterior plane was used on this first appliance to avoid delays at achieving overbite reduction during canine retraction. The second appliance was used to complete canine retraction (canines tend to follow the buccal segments and therefore require very little movement) prior to overjet reduction.

With this appliance tubes were soldered directly to the molar clasps because of the difficulty of including premolar clasps without interfering with the labial retractor. The clasps generally survive without fracture, probably because the headgear wear is reduced to provide only extraoral anchorage during this second phase of treatment.

COMMENTS ON TREATMENT

As the tracing reveals, growth was favourable and half the overjet reduction was obtained by mandibular forward growth. This was reflected by a 4.5 mm reduction of overjet occurring during the first phase of treatment, which lasted only 4 months. By this time the upper second molars were erupting very distally inclined and rather buccally displaced and it was decided that these should be removed. No canine retraction was required and the overjet reduction took only a further 4 months with the second appliance.

The oral hygiene had remained very poor during treatment and considerable palatal hyperplasia had resulted. In view of this and because of a desire to obtain a better buccal occlusion but at the same time to maintain retention until the growth spurt had ceased, a functional appliance of the activator type was employed as a retainer. This was worn at night for a further 6 months.

The models shown were taken at the end of retention. The case was followed up for 2 years but the patient objected to further models being taken. The overjet increased slightly in the first year and remained stable thereafter at 5 mm.

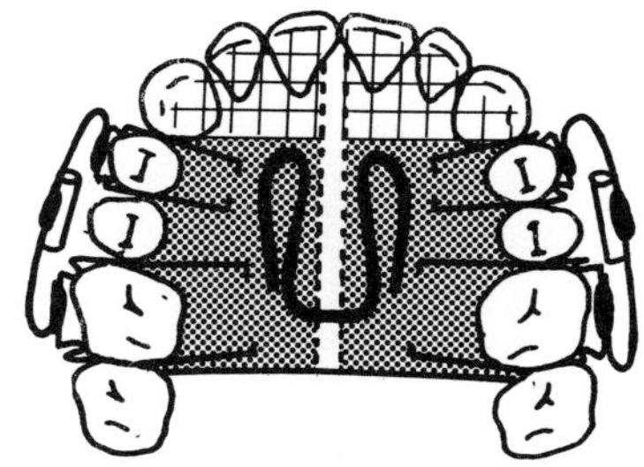

Appliance 1

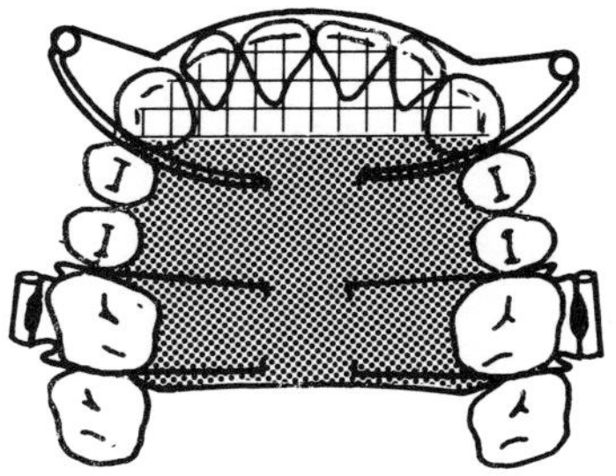

Appliance 2

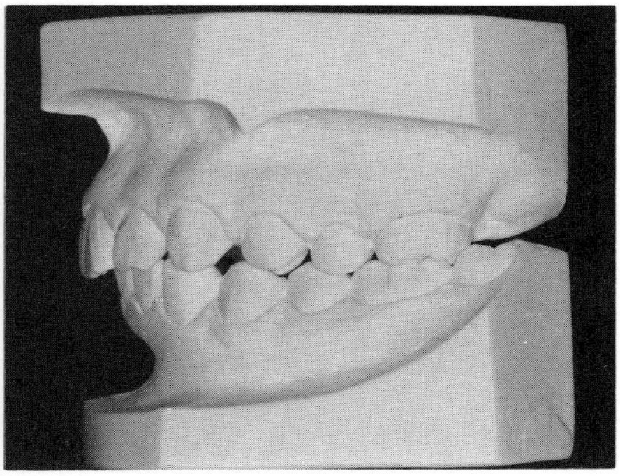

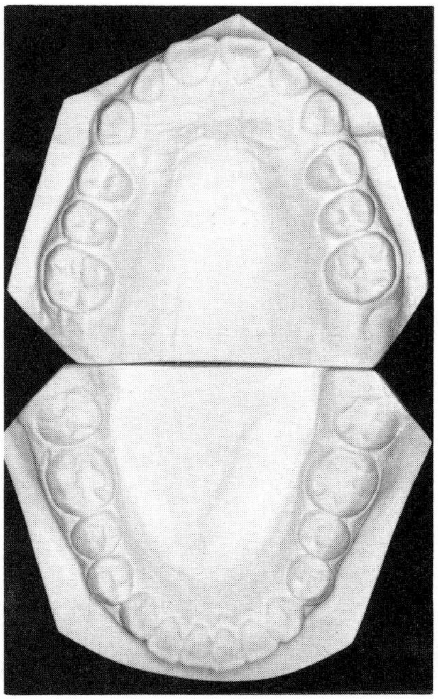

Further reading

It is to be hoped that the use of the book will at least encourage those who graduated some time ago to read some of the more recent textbooks. We suggest that the following might be consulted:

Houston W J B, Isaacson K G (1982). *Orthodontic Treatment with Removable Appliances* 2nd edn. Bristol: Wright.

Isaacson K G, Reed R T, Stephens C D (1989), *Functional Orthodontic Appliances*. Oxford: Blackwell Scientific.

Isaacson K G, Williams J K (1984). *An Introduction to Fixed Appliances* 3rd edn. Bristol: Wright.

Mills J R E (1987). *The Principles and Practice of Orthodontics* 2nd edn. Edinburgh: Churchill Livingstone.

Shaw W C (ed) (in preparation). *The Occlusion in Health and Disease.* Oxford: Heinemann Medical.

Index

The twenty treatment planning exercises
Pre-treatment records, 24–63
Case assessments, 66–85
Treatment plans and results, including a commentary on treatment carried out, 88–127

Users are asked to resist the temptation to check their findings as they go along, and to complete each section of a case before proceeding to the next.